In the Blink of an Eye

Andrew W. Artenstein, M.D.

In the Blink of an Eye

The Deadly Story of Epidemic Meningitis

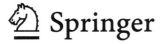 Springer

Andrew W. Artenstein, M.D.
Chair, Department of Medicine
Baystate Health
Springfield, MA, USA

ISBN 978-1-4614-4844-0   ISBN 978-1-4614-4845-7 (eBook)
DOI 10.1007/978-1-4614-4845-7
Springer New York Heidelberg Dordrecht London

Library of Congress Control Number: 2012948987

Printed on acid-free paper

Springer is part of Springer Science+Business Media (www.springer.com)

To my wife, Debbie, who listened—and shared my excitement—as the story unfolded and became a part of our life.
She is my greatest supporter, best friend, and the love of my life.

About the Author

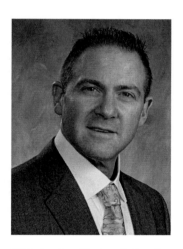

Andrew W. Artenstein, MD is the Chair of the Department of Medicine for Baystate Health System in Springfield, Massachusetts. Prior to this, he was the Physician-in-Chief and the Founding Director of the Center for Biodefense and Emerging Pathogens at Memorial Hospital of Rhode Island and Professor of Medicine and Health Services, Policy and Practice at The Warren Alpert Medical School of Brown University. He is an infectious diseases physician who is actively engaged in the arenas of research, medical education, clinical medicine, and public health. He is the author of more than 80 articles and book chapters on subjects related to infectious diseases, vaccines, biodefense, and medical history. He is the editor and lead author of *Vaccines: A Biography*, a history of vaccines and vaccinology.

Contents

Chapter 1
Origins

When the first warm breezes of April blow in from Buzzard's Bay, the South End of New Bedford, near the elbow of the Massachusetts coast as it extends eastward out to Cape Cod, changes character entirely. Not that the fast-food places, convenience stores, double-decker tenements, or boarded-up businesses transform magically into some sort of suburban Valhalla, but the change of season at least encourages people to go out on the streets and makes everything seem a little brighter.

Like many other small to mid-sized New England cities, New Bedford was once a vibrant manufacturing center. From the whaling industry of the eighteenth and early nineteenth centuries to the textile industry of the latter portion of the nineteenth and first half of the twentieth centuries, the city thrived. But New Bedford, like Fall River, Taunton, Lawrence, Lowell, Nashua, New Haven, Pawtucket, and other bygone industrial cities of the northeastern United States, has been down on its luck since the exodus of manufacturing jobs to the cheaper southern states and overseas. That, coupled with the devastation wrought by the influx of heroin and then crack cocaine in the 1970s and 1980s, respectively, virtually ensured the cumulative, continuous cycle of poverty that has gripped the population there ever since. Nonetheless, despite all the despair, the transition from winter to spring always brings the promise of a new beginning.

The first sign that change is afoot can be seen on the ball fields and playgrounds. Children and teenagers emerge as if responding to an unseen force. Impromptu baseball games appear, despite the nearly unusable, muddy infields and the swamp-like outfields caused by the recently melted snows and months of sun deprivation. The basketball courts, too, are beehives of activity, with groups of kids trying to make up for the time lost to the long, exhausting New England winter.

Michael Gomes, a reserve forward on the local high school basketball team, had seen little playing time during his sophomore season that ended when they lost in the first round of the state tournament in March. Although he had been good enough to make the varsity team, he knew that it would take an entire off-season of work to reach his goal of being a starter next year. It was for this reason that he decided to

A.W. Artenstein, *In the Blink of an Eye: The Deadly Story of Epidemic Meningitis*, DOI 10.1007/978-1-4614-4845-7_1, © Springer Science+Business Media New York 2013

try to forget about the throbbing ache in his head and take advantage of the first decent day of the early spring to join a pick-up game with some of the older, neighborhood boys at the city courts.

He had awakened with a dull pain over the back of his head and neck and assumed that he had slept in an unusual position, causing muscle spasms. He took Advil, an anti-inflammatory medicine that had always worked for aches, pains, and the occasional headache he had suffered in the past. This seemed to have alleviated the pain somewhat and allowed him to sleep for a few extra hours. But he still had the headache when he woke up; he was not a kid who usually got headaches.

During the pick-up game, Michael felt cold, something distinctly unusual as he was usually too warm during games. He put on a sweatshirt even though the other players were all in either T-shirts or bare-chested. Nonetheless, the game helped him forget about his headache temporarily. He played reasonably well and felt that it was a pretty good start to what would be a busy spring and summer of playing. On the short walk home around noon, he felt the sudden urge to vomit and did so on the sidewalk; he had never done that before. The headache was back in full force, throbbing in the back of his head. The sunlight bothered his eyes and made the headache seem worse. He found it difficult to bend his neck or turn from side to side. When he got home, he went straight to his bedroom, closed the shades, turned off the lights, and tried to sleep, hoping that he would feel better after a few hours.

When his mother came home from work at 5 o'clock, she went into Michael's room, surprised to find him asleep in his bed at this hour of the day. When she could not awaken him, only getting moans and unintelligible words in response to shaking him and shouting his name, she knew that something was wrong and called 9-1-1 for help. At the hospital's emergency room, the nurses found Michael to have a high fever, a stiff, rigid neck, and when they removed his clothes, the doctors observed faint, purplish spots on his skin around the area of the elastic waistband of his gym shorts; a few areas on his belly looked like small bruises. He seemed to be going in and out of consciousness; when arousable, he would try to answer their questions, but for the most part his answers did not make any sense. He was becoming increasingly agitated.

Michael's mother gave permission for them to perform a spinal tap, a test in which a needle is inserted into the space between the bones of the lower back in order to take a sample of the fluid that surrounds the spinal cord and brain. The fluid the doctors removed, normally thin and crystal clear, was cloudy, white, and thick. Michael had pyogenic meningitis, a bacterial infection that affects the tissues—the meninges—that cover the brain and spinal cord in the central nervous system. Despite the best efforts of modern medicine and powerful treatments that were brought to bear in the case of Michael Gomes, he died within 24 hours. A healthy, 16-year-old boy playing basketball with friends one day, gone the next—in the blink of an eye—another victim of a devastating disease that kills or permanently disables many thousands of individuals worldwide each year in its sporadic—episodic— form and has the potential to kill orders of magnitude more than that in its epidemic form. The disease has earned its status as one of the most dreaded contagious diseases of nature.

Outbreaks of infectious diseases were probably not a major concern of our earliest ancestors. The intimate, complex relationship between human beings and infectious diseases occurred only as a consequence of human social evolution. Early humans lived in small, scattered bands of hunter-gatherers; their primary concern was their own survival. And this essentially meant two things: figuring out where their next meal would come from while at the same time avoiding becoming someone else's meal or the unfortunate victim of some other deadly accident.

The relatively short life spans of our earliest ancestors were the result of starvation, predation, environmental exposures, and lethal trauma rather than the result of epidemic infections.[1] Infectious illnesses can only flourish in human groups when they can be passed from one member to another—a chain of transmission. Hence, infectious diseases are also known as "transmissible" or "communicable" illnesses. Because early humans traveled and lived in only small groups, the chain was, by definition, a short one. It could neither support the persistence nor the amplification of infection. Thus, the spread of any infectious disease would have been extinguished along with its human hosts—preventing the development of epidemics.

It was only with the advent of food-producing, large, dense, immobile, agricultural societies that conditions were created in which epidemics of infectious diseases could be maintained.[1] Social urbanization created a climate in which populations increased exponentially; the result—societies evolved into complex structures and became self-sustaining. Such societies not only developed governing organizations and well-defined social strata, but they also provided the ideal breeding ground for germs. Contagious infections flourished under such conditions. Disease transmission was facilitated through the crowded, unsanitary living conditions that characterized ancient societies, and their epidemic potential became magnified. It should therefore come as no surprise that infections such as smallpox, plague, tuberculosis, dysentery, and pneumonia were primarily responsible for the limited life expectancy and death of a significant proportion of the population in early modern Europe.[2]

One of the most significant 'episodes' in the development of human societies occurred nearly 10,000 years ago when inhabitants of the Fertile Crescent, in what is the modern-day Middle East, first successfully domesticated plants and animals. These actions benefited humans in a variety of important ways—and altered our collective fate. Domestication reduced the risk of starvation by providing a ready and regenerative supply of protein and other necessary nutrients. With the improved nutritional status of women, fecundity rates steadily rose, leading to favorable and sustained effects on childbearing and thus promoting the further growth of communities. Domestication of animals also provided humans with easily accessible sources of transportation and work. The cultivation of crops led to the establishment of permanent housing close to agricultural fields and livestock. Each of these factors improved the odds of survival of the human species.

But the successful domestication of animals was accompanied by a significant downside; the increasing proximity of humans to animals had the unintended effect of exposing humans to infectious diseases of animals—"zoonoses." Although crossing the species barrier is a difficult process for bacteria, viruses, parasites, and other infection-causing "pathogens," once accomplished, the germs enjoy unfettered access to a new host species, unencumbered by any of their new host's preexisting immunologic experiences. This can set the stage for epidemic diseases. Ancient examples abound: camelpox in domesticated camels became human smallpox, the greatest disease scourge of all time; bovine rinderpest became epidemic human measles; bovine tuberculosis became human tuberculosis, still a problem to this day; swine influenza became human influenza; and so on. More recent historical examples include the cross-species adaptation of human immunodeficiency virus type 1 (HIV-1) from simian immunodeficiency virus (SIV) of nonhuman primates—monkeys;[3] spongiform encephalopathy from sheep to cattle and on to humans as mad cow disease;[4] avian influenza from water fowl to humans through stops in chickens and pigs;[5] and severe acute respiratory disease (SARS) from civet cats to humans.[6]

The events of 10,000 years ago put humans on a path of accelerated social evolution. Adaptation from a nomadic, hunter-gather existence to a stable agrarian society with ample food supplies spawned a massive population explosion. A division of labor ensued resulting in the blossoming of civilization: science, innovation, government, and the arts.[1] But the gains in terms of civilized society were not without consequences with regard to disease—and infectious diseases reaped the benefits. The rapid expansion of densely populated, human communities with their attendant poor sanitation, absent sewage disposal, proximity to domesticated animals, and lack of understanding about the spread of contagious diseases created favorable conditions for outbreaks of infectious diseases—a pattern that continues unabated today in many parts of the world.

Other elements in the transmission of disease also acquired importance as human societies evolved. Rats, mice, and their rodent cousins, emboldened by feeding upon the enormous amounts of refuse generated by large, urban population centers, became efficient reservoirs—sources of germs—and vectors—transmission vehicles—for infections such as epidemic typhus and plague. Large groups of humans living in stable, agrarian communities provided a fertile environment for the airborne transmission of respiratory pathogens and also for the exchange of sexually transmitted infections—such as gonorrhea and syphilis—between intimate partners.[7] Human infectious diseases became a part of the fabric of civilization.

Epidemic infectious diseases in ancient cultures were believed to be of divine etiology.[2, 8] Many had a profound effect upon civilizations. Ancient Greek hegemony never recovered from the devastation wrought by the plague of Athens that began in 430 BC—early in the Peloponnesian War—and was caused by measles or perhaps another highly contagious infectious disease.[9] The Antonine plague of 165–169 AD, likely due to smallpox, originated in the eastern reaches of the Roman Empire—modern-day Iraq—before it spread widely and played a significant role in the inexorable decline of that superpower.[10]

Recurring pandemics—epidemics occurring over broad geographic areas—and sporadic—episodic—focal outbreaks of infectious diseases have played important roles in shaping the course of human history.[1, 11, 12] The Justinian plague of 541–544 AD was simply the opening salvo in 11 bubonic and pneumonic plague epidemics that disseminated and resurged in cycles throughout the known world of that time over a period of two centuries.[2, 13] It has been estimated that up to fifty percent of the population perished, contributing to major sociopolitical changes in the Byzantine Empire and leading Europe into the Middle Ages.[14]

Plague—the "Black Death"—arrived again in Sicily in 1347 via the trade routes from Asia, devastating the population of Europe and likely changing the course of history through its impact on geopolitics, armies, medieval commerce, and almost all aspects of daily and cultural life.[1, 15] The impact of the epidemic in Europe may have extended to the very core of humans—their genetic structure—altering the predisposition to future infectious diseases in that population via gene mutations, themselves driven by the selective pressure to evolve and thus survive in the face of the plague.[16]

Repeated exposure to infections had other effects as well. It allowed humans to develop highly evolved immune systems—defensive weapons in the battle against germs—that became a major advantage for survival. Because communicable diseases were so prevalent, European societies became immunologically experienced to many pathogens; their body's defense mechanisms learned how to fight off germs that they had previously encountered. With each round of epidemic infection—measles, smallpox, plague, or other scourge—enlightened observers had noted the phenomenon of "resistance" to sickness upon reexposure to the same disease process. Hence, over time, those who had been previously exposed were able to resist many infectious diseases—if they survived the first encounter. These infections, therefore, became a part of society's morbid landscape, causing episodic eruptions of disease in nonimmune people but no longer carrying the same explosive mortality for the whole community.[2]

However, circumstances were entirely different when populations were exposed to infectious germs for the first time. In this setting, some pathogens behaved differently—and particularly badly. Many infections were much more aggressive—deadly—when they encountered populations without any previous exposure to the germ. Immunologically naïve societies were therefore much more vulnerable as compared to immunologically experienced ones.[17]

The historical record is replete with vivid examples of the consequences of an infectious germ entering a population that had not previously experienced its wrath. Columbus' first voyage across the Atlantic in 1492 unleashed Europe's repertoire of epidemic infectious diseases on the immunologically virginal population of the New World—a dynamic that continued with successive Old World incursions into the Americas over the next 150 years. Indigenous populations were decimated as smallpox epidemics ravaged the island of Hispaniola in the first quarter of the sixteenth century, reducing the population by more than ninety five percent.[18]

Other Native American societies of the Caribbean basin and later Mexico, Guatemala, and Brazil fell victim to multiple infections imported from the Old World: dysentery, influenza, malaria, and measles among them. With epidemic smallpox in tow, introduced by Spanish forces rampaging through the Indian population of central Mexico, Hernán Cortés was able to easily subjugate the immense Aztec Empire with fewer than five hundred men in 1521.[18, 19] His compatriot, Francisco Pizarro, was the beneficiary of a similar result against the Incas in Peru a decade later.[19]

An analogous fate was met by other immunologically naïve populations when novel diseases were introduced via friendly or hostile visitors from areas known to harbor the pathogens. Yellow fever virus entered the New World through the transatlantic slave trade from Africa.[20] It caused recurrent, highly lethal epidemics in coastal areas of the Americas from the seventeenth century through the early part of the twentieth century. In Philadelphia, the disease killed ten percent of the city's population in 1793.[21] A decade later yellow fever decimated Napoleon's expeditionary forces in Haiti, forcing the "Little Corporal" to abandon his imperial plans for the Americas and to sell the Louisiana Territory to the newly independent United States.[20] A century later the disease again altered history by driving the French out of the Panama Canal development process and later almost derailing the American effort there.[22] Measles, imported into the isolated Faroe Islands in the North Atlantic by an infected carpenter in1846, caused an epidemic that infected nearly eighty percent of the population within six months.[23]

Within their evolutionary framework, epidemic infectious diseases of numerous varieties were well established in human society by the second millennium. Informed by the burgeoning of scientific thought of the eighteenth century's Age of Enlightenment, hypotheses were beginning to be formulated regarding transmissible infectious diseases and their causative agents. By the nineteenth century, scientific knowledge and technology had developed to such an extent that some of these theories could finally be formally tested—and either confirmed or refuted. The lethal infection that killed young Michael Gomes would be among those whose mystery would begin to be unraveled.

Chapter 2
The Art and Science of Germs

As human civilizations began to flourish, so did the infectious diseases that afflicted them. Over time, an understanding of these contagious sicknesses gradually developed, but not as rapidly as developments in other areas of medicine. Despite major advances in science and medicine that occurred in the first and early second millennia AD in China, India, Persia, and the Islamic world, and more accelerated developments that followed during The Renaissance and the Age of Enlightenment, the specific causes of infectious illnesses defied explanation and remained in the realm of the occult. The Franciscan monk, Roger Bacon, had originally described the fundamental principles of the scientific method in 1269, stressing the formulation of hypotheses based on observations from nature and the primacy of experimentation to confirm such hypotheses. Yet, he and his contemporaries lacked the tools and techniques to adequately study events that could not be observed by the human eye; contagious diseases fell into this category. This remained the major impediment to the advancement of the discipline over the ensuing 400 years.

To the ancients and their descendants well into the second millennium, the cause of infections had been variously ascribed to divine punishment for sins and other human failings; the results of poor hygiene; and the consequences of changes in climate or atmospheric conditions related to cosmic activities—the concept of "bad air" or "miasma".[1] Although the causes of infections were poorly understood, their contagious nature had been well documented. The Old Testament contains several references—and suggested remedies—regarding contagion.[2] The kosher food laws from *Leviticus* may have represented one such remedy, borne out of health concerns as much as anything else. However, the first organized view that microscopic germs may be causes of disease was not articulated until the sixteenth century.

Using his remarkable powers of observation and knowledge of epidemics, the Italian physician Girolamo Fracastoro, also known as Hieronymus Fracastorius, culminated sixteen years of research in 1546 with the publication of "*de Contagione*," a treatise that represented the first scientific discussion of the concepts of germs, contagion, transmission, and their application to a variety of infectious diseases. In it he prophetically surmised that tiny, free-living germs exist in nature and are capable of causing disease. Despite being invisible to human eyes, these organisms could

A.W. Artenstein, *In the Blink of an Eye: The Deadly Story of Epidemic Meningitis*, DOI 10.1007/978-1-4614-4845-7_2, © Springer Science+Business Media New York 2013

be transmitted from person to person directly or via inanimate object intermediaries, thereby spreading illness between people.[3]

Although penned a century before microscopic germs would actually be seen, Fracastorius' work remains a landmark of clarity in the field. But it was not his most popular work; he is perhaps best known for naming and characterizing syphilis, disparagingly referred to as "the French Sickness" by the Italians and as "the Italian Disease" by the French. In "*Syphilis sive Morbus Gallicus*," written years before his treatise on contagion, he painted in poetic verse a remarkably accurate, detailed picture of the clinical consequences of the "great masquerader"—the disease that mimicked countless others.[4]

More than one hundred years after Fracastorius, the "seeds of disease" were visualized for the first time. Although he did not invent the microscope—that feat having been accomplished late in the sixteenth or early in the seventeenth century— Antony van Leeuwenhoek became the first to use a simple version of the device to actually identify microorganisms, the germs that he likened to "little animals" or "animalcules" in 1676. Leeuwenhoek, a Dutch textile merchant and self-taught amateur scientist, had taken an interest in creating magnifying lenses and building microscopes. He apparently used these to make an enormous variety of observations on natural phenomena, which he duly reported to the most important scientific body of the time—the newly formed Royal Society of London.

In his most famous, 18th letter to the Royal Society, Leeuwenhoek described the little creatures he saw under his microscopes in a sample of rain water left standing for four days, in river water from his hometown of Delft, in well water from his courtyard, in seawater, and in water that he infused with fresh peppercorns, cloves, nutmeg, and ginger.[5] Despite the likelihood that most of the "animalcules" he noted in these initial observations were not bacteria but protozoa, a subkingdom of microorganisms that are significantly larger in size and more complex in function than bacteria, his findings were still revolutionary. Seven years later, Leeuwenhoek observed and characterized with astonishing accuracy a variety of morphological forms of bacteria found in samples obtained from teeth scrapings of children and adults, including his own.

Although Leeuwenhoek confirmed Fracastoro's sixteenth century hypothesis,[6] and his own findings were subsequently validated by others, the critical significance of these tiny forms to human health would not be fully appreciated until almost 200 years later when an industrial chemist in Paris named Louis Pasteur and subsequently a military physician named Robert Koch in Berlin successfully cultured bacterial organisms from diseased tissues, thus confirming the "germ theory" of disease causation and ushering in the era of modern medical microbiology. Meanwhile, in the time period between Leeuwenhoek and Pasteur, multiple iterations, variations, and opposing views regarding whether germs caused disease were promulgated and debated in enlightened society.[7] Definitive proof of such theories still awaited the discovery of scientific tools enabling their validation; nonetheless, empiric evidence supporting the concept that microscopic germs caused infectious diseases mounted dramatically with the seminal observations of two European physicians and a holy botanist in the mid-nineteenth century.

By the mid-1800s, childbed or puerperal fever, originally described by the great Hippocrates in his famous *Corpus*, was well recognized as a highly mortal and all too common complication of obstetrical care on hospital maternity wards. This illness, occurring within days of delivery, resulted from intrauterine infection leading to profound inflammation of the uterus and contiguous organs in the female abdomen and pelvis and, in many cases, to the rapid spread of infection via the bloodstream—leading to death of the mother. While childbed fever was not then known to be an overwhelming bacterial infection as it is today, it was felt by some in the medical profession to be a contagious illness, and it was the most common cause of maternal mortality at the time. The rising number and growth of hospitals that accompanied nascent industrialization in Europe in the eighteenth and nineteenth centuries meant that more women were giving birth on maternity wards; a greater concentration of postpartum women translated to more opportunities for lethal outbreaks of childbed fever.

Allgemeine Krankenhaus—Vienna General Hospital with its associated Lying-in or obstetrical hospital—opened in 1784. Like other such hospitals of the time, it became a major venue for the medical care of society's poor and served an important role in providing a training ground for young men seeking to become physicians. The Lying-in hospital comprised two obstetrical services that alternated admissions on a daily basis: the First Division, operated by physicians and medical students, and the Second, run by midwives. Because of the need to teach the medical students, more internal examinations were performed on each pregnant woman on the First Division. In the mid-1840s, childbed fever was rampant in the hospital; more than fifteen percent of postpartum women on the First Division succumbed to childbed fever, a figure nearly tenfold higher than that of women on the Second, midwife-operated Division. To Ignác Semmelweis, a young Hungarian obstetrician and newly appointed assistant to the head of the Lying-in hospital, finding the cause of the illness involved solving the riddle of the discrepancy between Divisions. The results of his epidemiologic and pathologic investigation would eventually advance the germ theory of disease causation.[8]

The autopsy—dissection of the dead—was a critically important component of nineteenth century medicine and medical education. It was the primary tool used to teach anatomy and pathology to medical students, and in the absence of X-rays and other techniques of imaging the internal body during life, it represented the best opportunity to make identifiable links between altered anatomy—structure—and clinical manifestations of diseases. Unlike medicine of today, where autopsies have become an uncommon event and medical trainees rarely get the chance to learn from the dead, these procedures were routinely performed in European hospitals, especially those in the German-speaking world. Nowhere was this more highly valued than at the Allgemeine Krankenhaus and its Lying-in hospital. Nearly every woman who died of puerperal fever underwent an autopsy, generally by the same groups of doctors and medical students that moved continuously between the autopsy room and the wards of the First Division to examine expectant mothers and perform deliveries. And therein proved to be a clue that allowed Semmelweis to unravel the epidemiologic mystery behind the cause of childbed fever.

Semmelweis made several observations in conjunction with the aforementioned initial one in 1847 that led him to suspect a germ as the cause of the illness that plagued the First Division. He noted that in some cases, the infant delivered of a woman with childbed fever succumbed to a similar illness, suggesting a communicable cause. This idea received further credence by another event, the death of a respected pathologist at the institution, Professor Kolletschka, due to an overwhelming infection resulting from an accidental blade injury during an autopsy; the findings on Kolletschka's autopsy appeared similar to those of the victims of childbed fever. Semmelweis recognized that the putrid odor associated with women dying of puerperal fever was similar to that emanating from corpses during autopsies and noted that the malodorous smell from the corpses was also found on the hands of the doctors performing the procedures. Additionally, he observed that the attending physicians and medical students did not generally wash their hands after leaving the autopsy room to see their pregnant patients or after attending to patients with other infections. Finally, he observed that the death rate from puerperal fever declined significantly when the medical students were on vacation and no autopsies were being performed. Synthesizing this information, Semmelweis correctly hypothesized that some form of "putrid matter" must be carried on the hands of physicians and students during their rounds between the autopsy and birthing tables or between patients on the wards, and that this might be transmitted to pregnant women resulting in a highly lethal peripartum illness.[9]

To his great credit, Semmelweis made these observations without the benefit of formal training in microbiology; in fact, the discipline did not exist at the time. The idea that invisible germs could be responsible for illness—the "germ theory of disease"—was neither taught in medical schools nor accepted as truth. This situation would not change until the work of Pasteur and his disciples became widely accepted later in the nineteenth century. But for a variety of reasons, some of which were deeply ingrained personality flaws, he failed to follow-up his astute epidemiological observations with the next logical steps expected of the medical scientist and therefore never sought proof, possible with the state of microscopy at the time, that "animalcules" were present in the "putrid matter"—pus—found in the autopsied abdominal and pelvic cavities of childbed fever victims. There were no rigorous laboratory experiments that would have proved his hypothesis, and despite multiple opportunities and the well-intentioned urging of his proponents, no published manuscript emerged to explain his reasoning and thought process. His views on puerperal fever, correct though they turned out to be, also flew in the face of his chain of command at the hospital. By failing to convincingly demonstrate the merits of his ideas to the medical staff, Semmelweis became alienated and marginalized.

To be sure, this doctrine of Semmelweis was provocative and went against the grain of the old guard at the University of Vienna and elsewhere among the hallowed halls of academic medicine in Europe. What's more, it directly implicated physicians as vectors in the transmission of a deadly disease to their patients. This, perhaps more than any other element in his controversial hypothesis, rankled the medical establishment. Historically, innovative ideas that contradict prevailing wisdom are vulnerable to immediate rejection. Semmelweis' views were unpopular and placed him squarely apart from his professional colleagues; he did little to try to diffuse the situation, in fact he made it worse. His oratory and literary skills in German were inadequate, making it difficult to effectively communicate his ideas to colleagues in Vienna.[10] Additionally, his dogmatic and inflexible style, worsening with every passing year, further alienated him from his peers.

While he never performed the scientific experiments to prove his hypothesis, he did empirically institute a strict hand-washing requirement for all medical students and faculty—using a dilute chloride lime solution that was known to remove the odor from putrid materials—before patient contact. With this measure alone, Semmelweis demonstrated a dramatic decline in the incidence of childbed fever and maternal mortality on the First Division. Nonetheless, he found himself out of a job in academic medicine and back in his native Hungary within short order.

It took Semmelweis until 1861 to publish the definitive review of his investigations; what emerged was a rambling, incoherent report that convinced few of his skeptics and only further diminished his standing among his peers. He countered with a series of harsh diatribes against his critics, essentially accusing his fellow physicians of killing their patients through negligence. Compounding his lack of interpersonal and communication skills, Semmelweis was operating during a moment of great geopolitical turmoil, a world in which every action and reaction was riddled with political overtones and nationalistic biases. By 1848, the concept of revolution was spreading throughout Europe; within the Hapsburg Empire, of which Austria and Hungary were parts, the tenuous Dual Monarchy was teetering under the separatist demands of Hungarian nationalists. As a result, a wave of national conservatism gripped Austria. Semmelweis, a foreigner with radical and unpopular ideas about infection control, was already somewhat of a pariah among the medical community there and was caught in the vise and ostracized. Back in Hungary his behavior became increasingly erratic resulting in his involuntary commitment to an insane asylum, where he died unexpectedly under suspicious circumstances, apparently and ironically secondary to an overwhelming bacterial infection related to traumatic injuries—possibly a result of beatings.

While Semmelweis was making his observations on Vienna's hospital wards, John Snow, a prominent London physician, was also accumulating epidemiologic evidence of microorganisms as causes of human illness in a community outbreak of a deadly diarrheal disease. Massive population expansion and concentration into overcrowded urban areas had occurred in Europe throughout the nineteenth century as a result of industrialization. Nowhere was this more evident than in London. Standards of hygiene and sanitary practices in Victorian London were either poor or nonexistent. The flush toilet, patented in 1819, was not yet in widespread use. The effluent from water closets and public privies was simply deposited into local rivers; the largest and most important—the Thames—was the primary source of drinking water for the city and was essentially converted into an open sewer.

Cholera, a diarrheal scourge once described as "the disease that begins where other diseases end—with death," became a worldwide threat in the early part of the nineteenth century as it traversed the globe killing hundreds of thousands in Asia, Africa, and Europe.[11] Large urban outbreaks of cholera terrorized Britain in 1831 and again in the late 1840s. In 1849, Snow published a pamphlet in which he challenged the prevailing theory that cholera resulted from bad air—"miasma"— and instead speculated that it was waterborne.[12] Another outbreak in 1854 in his own South London neighborhood provided the grand experiment by which to test his alternative hypothesis.

Snow carefully mapped the incident cases of cholera among the residents of South London and noted their proximity to public water-drawing sites. Using the rudimentary, newly minted morbidity and mortality statistics of the era, he noted that the highest incidence of disease was clustered around the corner of Broad and Cambridge Streets, a public pumping station for drinking water. The water intake for this pump was drawn from a location just downstream of a large sewer effluent from London in the Thames River. Through interviews of cases and contacts and statistical assessments—"shoe-leather" epidemiologic methods that would become standard fare for future outbreak investigators but were novel at the time—Snow deduced that the infection was transmitted by contaminated water obtained from the Broad Street pump. As a result of his evidence, the handle was removed from the Broad Street pump forcing local residents to seek water from other pumping stations. The epidemic, probably already waning, was halted.[13]

The circumstances provided compelling evidence in favor of Snow's transmission hypothesis; he is appropriately credited as the founding father of the field of epidemiology based on this work. However, like Semmelweis, Snow never obtained definitive microbiologic proof that germs in the drinking water were actually the cause of the epidemic. It would take another 30 years, well into the period of rapid microbiological discovery, before Robert Koch and his colleagues finally isolated *Vibrio cholerae*, the etiologic agent of this dread disease.[12, 14] Nonetheless, evidence in favor of the germ theory continued to mount at mid century. However, the most compelling clue would not derive from an outbreak of human disease but from a simple root vegetable rotting in the fields of Ireland.

Around the same time that Semmelweis and Snow were making their seminal observations among Vienna's parturient women and South London's poor, respectively, Reverend Miles J. Berkeley, English cleric and amateur plant taxonomist, was making his on rotting potatoes. His findings would represent another, incremental step forward for the germ theory of disease.

Outbreaks of a rotting disease had ravaged the crop in parts of the United States and Canada in the early 1840s and by 1845, acting in synergy with a particularly cold, rainy period, these began destroying almost the entire Irish potato crop over the next few years. Berkeley was a mycologist—an expert on the fungi that accounted for the fuzzy, colorful mold on old bread and the slippery growths on the moist floor of the forest. While studying black spots on potato leaves and tubers in 1846, he noted the unmistakable presence of microscopic mold elements on all diseased plants. This simple observation—the "potato blight"—would herald, over the next decade, the collapse of Irish society, leading to the death of one million and the mass emigration of at least another million of their countrymen from their homeland—never to return.[14, 15]

Although the potato blight was epidemic throughout Europe at the time, the disease disproportionately affected Irish society. Irish soil was poorly tolerant of other crops, making the potato the dietary staple and primary source of protein and carbohydrate for that country's poor and working class, a significant swath of the population. Additionally, British subjugation of Ireland ensured a cycle of dependency on this vegetable as a source of income based on its forced exportation.

As with others, Semmelweis and Snow included, whose theories were contrary to prevailing wisdom, the scientific community did not immediately embrace Berkeley's observations. It was generally accepted at the time that the blight, like childbed fever and cholera, was due to cold and damp "miasma"—bad air (interestingly, the cold and moist environmental conditions likely favored the dissemination of the fungus). Berkeley demonstrated only the association of mold elements with the potato disease, never providing the definitive experimental confirmation.[16] But in 1861, the same year that Semmelweis finally wrote his now famous if fatally flawed paper on puerperal fever and shortly before the validity of the germ theory of disease was conclusively demonstrated in Paris, Anton de Bary, a German plant pathologist and mycologist, conclusively proved that the etiology of potato blight was in fact a fungus. He named it *Phytophthora infestans*—"the plant destroyer"—and had proven its causal role by essentially following the same lines of scientific reasoning that would set the standard for microbial causation two decades later in a Berlin tuberculosis laboratory.

Despite the accumulating body of evidence favoring microbes as causes of disease, the actual inception of microbiology as a distinct science traditionally dates to 1857, when the great Louis Pasteur convincingly demonstrated that microorganisms were responsible for the fermentation of certain liquids. Up until that time, the most popular theory to explain a host of biological processes from the origins of life forms to putrefaction—the spoiling of organic materials—was "spontaneous generation." The latter concept was extrapolated to explain the origins of disease as well. Pasteur's work debunked spontaneous generation and showed instead that fermentation, spoiling, or contamination of organic substances was due to the presence of environmental microorganisms—not to some type of magical transformation. These investigations had the indirect effect of proving the germ theory of disease.

Using early prototype microscopes, Leeuwenhoek and his English contemporary Robert Hooke had clearly demonstrated the presence of unicellular protozoan and tiny bacterial organisms—the "little animalcules"—in the latter part of the seventeenth century.[17] Plant pathologists and mycologists had demonstrated the essential role of microorganisms as the cause of selected diseases of plants, including the potato blight. Yet by the middle of the nineteenth century, it was still unproven whether microorganisms could actually cause human diseases. Neither Semmelweis nor Snow had actually been able to conclusively demonstrate the connection. Moreover, even the mere presence of organisms in diseased tissues raised the inevitable question as to whether these organisms arose spontaneously from substances already present in devitalized material or whether they derived from exogenous sources and had to be implanted to cause disease.

The concept that living things derived from inanimate sources—the original theory of spontaneous generation—arose from Aristotle's attempts to reconcile his own observations with the philosophies of his ancient predecessors. Since nearly their first appearance on earth, humans have endeavored to understand the origins of life; the spontaneous generation of life from nonliving things, such as sea creatures from water, sea foam, and sand, or insects from soil, snow, or the sun, provided a convenient explanation of the incompletely understood, Ancient Greek world. This basic belief became the dogma of scholars and naturalists, and once accepted by the Christian Church in the early part of the second millennium, went essentially unchallenged for nearly 700 years.

In the same era that later spawned Leeuwenhoek's interest in microscopy, Francesco Redi, Italian physician, naturalist, and poet, became one of the first to experimentally challenge the doctrine of spontaneous generation. Based on the observation that maggots could be found on rotting meat and believing that these creatures derived from flies and not from the tissue itself, he sought to demonstrate this through a series of simple experiments involving dead snakes, eels, fish, and pieces of meat from various species of mammal placed in either open or closed containers.[18] While these seemed to prove that the generation of maggots required a living host, Redi sought to definitively determine whether these creatures arose from the food—spontaneous generation, or whether they were introduced exogenously.

In a final series of experiments, he included open containers that were covered with "fine Naples veil," a type of gauze netting that allowed the passage of air but not flies. The results of Redi's experiments were clear; open containers attracted flies that deposited their eggs, which developed into larvae—maggots—on the rotting meat. Containers covered with gauze developed maggots only on this surface, as the flies were attracted by the smell but could not land on the meat. No maggots were observed in the sealed containers. Life was not spontaneously generated; instead, it was life—in the form of insects in this case—that led to new life.

Changing deeply ingrained and widely accepted dogma does not occur quickly or painlessly. Despite Redi's findings, originally published in 1668 and disseminated widely in multiple translations throughout the late seventeenth century, the doctrine of spontaneous generation continued to gain adherents. The subject was widely debated and experimentally challenged by a number of scientists throughout the eighteenth and nineteenth centuries; the results of such experiments varied considerably, with some appearing to prove and others to dispel the hypothesis. Most of the variability, we now know, owed more to methodological design than to any real biological phenomena.[1] The germ theory of disease, postulating that illness arises from microscopic germs and the contrapuntal viewpoint to spontaneous generation, remained a minority opinion, despite having its renowned proponents—including Jakob Henle and Edwin Klebs—both celebrated German pathologists of the time and contemporaries of Pasteur.

The germ theory also had its influential detractors. One of its most vocal critics was Félix-Archimède Pouchet, Director of the Natural History Museum in Rouen, France, and a main advocate of spontaneous generation. Owing to the scientific and even political importance of the debate, the French Academy of Sciences offered a monetary prize in 1864 to the scientist who could provide definitive evidence to either prove or disprove the concept of spontaneous generation. Pasteur accepted the challenge and won the award through a series of elegant and carefully executed experiments that eliminated the possibility of spontaneous generation. Throughout the early 1860s, he studied the question in his laboratory in Paris, informed by his landmark work in the arena of fermentation, in which he discovered the source of the "ferment"—germs. Using various forms of glass flasks, some with drawn-out, swan-like necks that were either sealed or open, he showed that extreme heat or filtration of air and water could maintain organic materials in sterile conditions indefinitely without any microbial growth.[19] The microorganisms did not arise spontaneously within the materials; they were introduced from the environment and reproduced to create additional life forms.

Pasteur's simple, yet definitive experiments did not end the controversy over spontaneous generation, but they accelerated its demise. Techniques of sterilization—"Pasteurization"—of dairy products were soon introduced and undoubtedly saved millions of lives in the period that followed. Pasteur subsequently established the Institute that bears his name through a combination of private financing and public monies. The Pasteur Institute soon became an international center for microbiology, immunology, and medicine, in no small part due to the larger-than-life persona of Louis Pasteur himself. To this day, at 25 Rue De Doctor Roux—named after Pasteur's assistant and most famous disciple—portions of his laboratory remain preserved, along with the forever-sterile nutrient broth within the sealed, 150-year-old glass flasks. The great chemist himself still resides in the building; his crypt, walls adorned with artists' renderings of his professional achievements, is on the ground floor below his study and sitting room. On the ceiling, arching above Pasteur's tomb in inlaid, colorful mosaic tiles, rise the three Christian virtues—Faith, Hope, and Charity, to which the artist has added a fourth—Science—for that is the mother of all.

Shortly thereafter, the British surgeon Joseph Lister extended the great chemist's concepts to the clinical setting. Inferring, on the basis of Pasteur's revelations, that the "suppuration" and "decomposition" observed in infected surgical wounds resulted from "minute organisms suspended" in the air, he devised a method to "destroy the life of the floating particles".[20] Local farmers had discovered that carbolic acid decreased the fetid odor of their commonly used "night soil"—human excreta—fertilizer. Lister therefore used solutions of this chemical diluted with boiled linseed oil to form a paste, which he then mixed with lime to exert a "destructive influence upon low forms of life"—bacteria causing wound infections. His methods protected the wounds of patients with compound fractures against infections at the orthopedic infirmary in Glasgow, Scotland. Lister published his findings in 1867 in the widely read medical journal *The Lancet*.

The scientific community favorably received Lister's findings, and the use of sterile technique—antisepsis—in the care of surgical patients was rapidly adopted as an international standard.[21] This led directly to further advances with the use of chemical disinfectants to prevent wound infections and their use in maintaining the sterility of dressings, surgical instruments, and the hands of surgeons caring for injured patients.[22] Why was Lister's work accepted whereas that of his predecessors, most notably Semmelweis, had failed to sway the scientific and medical communities? At least in the very public case of Semmelweis, there are probably two important explanations. First, in the relatively brief span of time—two decades—after the Hungarian physician's work in Vienna, the germ theory of disease had garnered widespread acceptance, largely through the efforts of Pasteur.[23] Additionally, whereas Semmelweis presented his provocative findings as dogma—without following accepted scientific protocol of the scholarly presentation of data followed by the articulation of his thought processes in a highly visible, scientific publication—Lister was tactful, cautious in his presentation and was persuasive, not abrasive in his approach to the scientific community. Undoubtedly, politics played a role as well, given the highly charged, nationalistic climate in which Semmelweis—a foreigner—worked.

While Paris was fast becoming the center of research in the nascent field of microbiology, a country doctor from Prussia was beginning his scientific career essentially as a weekend hobby. Robert Koch studied medicine at the University at Göttingen where he came under the influence of the notable Professor of Anatomy and Pathology Jakob Henle—an early proponent of the germ theory of disease—and where he was indoctrinated in the importance of careful animal experimentation in understanding disease causation. In the 1870s, as a district medical officer in the Prussian town of Wollstein, Koch began his investigations into the etiology of anthrax, a disease of livestock that had a profoundly negative impact on the agricultural economy.[24] He identified anthrax bacilli in the blood of infected sheep and successfully transmitted the infection into healthy experimental animals. Using careful photomicroscopy and detailed drawings, he accurately depicted the life cycle of anthrax and the process of endospore formation. With the publication of this work in 1876, Koch became a major force in the fledgling field of microbiology.

Koch pioneered a number of laboratory techniques. He employed the use of the oil immersion microscope to study bacteria, vastly improving the visual resolution of these organisms; developed new methods for bacterial identification using special staining techniques; and invented procedures for the isolation of pure bacterial cultures on solid media. The ability to culture bacteria was facilitated by the use of agar as the solidifying agent on flat—"Petri"—dishes—named after their inventor and Koch assistant, Richard Petri—and still in common use today.[25]

While serving as a senior medical officer in the Imperial Health Office in Berlin in 1882, Koch discovered the microbial etiology of tuberculosis, perhaps the most important disease cause of death at the time, making his a household name.[26] Using his newly described differential staining, microscopy, and culture techniques, Koch isolated the causative agent, *Mycobacterium tuberculosis*, in pure culture.[27] It was in this context that he proposed a set of criteria that had to be satisfied to infer an etiologic role for a specific bacterial agent in a particular disease. These conditions that came to be known as "Koch's Postulates" rapidly became the gold standard upon which to judge evidence of microbial disease causation:[24]

- The pathogen accounts for the clinical and pathological features of the disease and must be found in every case in which the disease occurs
- The pathogen is not found in other diseases as a nonpathogen

- After being isolated from the body and repeatedly passed in pure culture, the pathogen can induce the disease in animal models
- The same pathogen must be reisolated from the experimental animal

Although refined over the years, these criteria are still valid to some extent today.

Koch, like Pasteur, surrounded himself with brilliant colleagues and collaborators and simultaneously attracted strong supporters and equally vocal detractors. Contemporary physicians who rejected the germ theory in favor of other theories of disease causation included Max von Pettenkoffer, the influential Munich hygienist, and the celebrated cellular pathologist Rudolf Virchow. Pettenkoffer espoused the "sanitation theory" of disease, widely supported by social liberals, that poor sanitation, unfavorable water, soil conditions, and damp weather generated miasma poisons that subsequently caused illness, primarily in socioeconomically disadvantaged populations. The cure for epidemics was therefore social progress and the elimination of poverty. Virchow, considered to be the founding father of cellular pathology and the most respected academic physician in Germany during Koch's era, remained an ardent opponent of the germ theory of infectious diseases. He never completely embraced Koch's discovery of the tubercle bacillus despite the overwhelming scientific evidence. However, Virchow did eventually capitulate to at least public acceptance of Koch's theories, returning to Berlin after The Pathological Institute was built for him on the grounds of Koch's Institute.[24, 28]

The conservative Prussian government in power in Berlin embraced the germ theory of disease largely because the fundamental premise was that communicable diseases were the consequences of exogenous microorganisms invading the body, circumstances that were largely independent of socioeconomics and therefore beyond governmental control. Infections could thus potentially be prevented without having to address all the ills of society. To show their appreciation, the Prussian Parliament supported Koch's work with lavish funding for the Koch Institute for Infectious Diseases, which opened its doors in Berlin in 1891.[24] The government's interests were not purely altruistic; these were fervently nationalistic times, and enmity was firmly entrenched between Germany and France after the French defeat in the Franco-Prussian War of 1870. When Koch's team succeeded in isolating the etiologic agent of cholera in Egypt after Pasteur's group had failed, the German government hailed it as proof of the superiority of German science over French science, and Koch returned to Berlin to a hero's procession.[24, 28]

Although from different cultures and harboring major differences in their styles and scientific approaches, Pasteur and Koch remain the two most influential figures in the history of microbiology. Through their work in the latter part of the nineteenth century, the germ theory of disease was confirmed and extended to identify a number of microbial causes of specific infectious diseases. The seeds had been sown; the fruits of discovery within the newly formed science of microbiology were ripe for the picking.

Chapter 3
A Singular Disease

The convergence of thought engendered by Pasteur's confirmation of the germ theory of disease, along with technological advances in the laboratory spearheaded by Koch, led to the premise by the latter part of the nineteenth century that many of the most notorious illnesses of the time could be ascribed a specific bacterial origin. Traditional rational empiricism—careful observations filtered through the lens of reason—that had been the guiding force of physicians through the ages could at last be wed to science.

The differentiation of individual diseases on a clinical basis had perhaps been most clearly articulated by Thomas Sydenham, the "father of English medicine," in the seventeenth century. His writings represent detailed observations on the clinical manifestations of a variety of well-recognized syndromes—many of them infectious in origin—of the time, including smallpox, plague, pertussis—"whooping cough"—and measles as well as descriptions of noninfectious entities such as gout—which the author himself suffered from for most of his adult life—and chorea, a bizarre movement disorder of the nervous system. Although classic and elegant, his observations were made prior to the application of the germ theory; in fact, Sydenham died just a decade after Leeuwenhoek's initial description of animalcules in rainwater. Thus, they were either silent on the etiology of these infectious maladies or, as in the case of smallpox—which he described in his famous book on the management of fevers as due to a type of "renovation" of the blood—were frankly wrong.[1]

The movement towards associating individual diseases with specific causes gained adherents in the eighteenth and early nineteenth centuries, largely through the study of pathological anatomy. It was this discipline that allowed practitioners of the art to correlate symptoms—what the patient complains of—and signs—findings on physical examination—with observations noted at the time of pathological examination, either following surgical extirpation of lesions or necropsy. As viewing techniques improved via better lenses and microscopes, gross findings—those visualized by the naked eye—could be correlated with observations made under the microscope, further enhancing the classification of disease processes. In this fashion, the knowledge gaps in medicine began to close as the tools with

A.W. Artenstein, *In the Blink of an Eye: The Deadly Story of Epidemic Meningitis*,
DOI 10.1007/978-1-4614-4845-7_3, © Springer Science+Business Media New York 2013

which to study the science improved. For infectious diseases, these tools derived from the experimental revelations that came from Paris and Berlin, centers of medicine of the era, and they would galvanize a flurry of microbiologic discovery.

Koch's approach in Berlin was more technically oriented than Pasteur's in Paris. After laying spontaneous generation to rest in favor of the germ theory, Pasteur, as we shall see later, turned his attention, following a series of serendipitous laboratory observations, to immunization—vaccination—as the principal means of protection against microbial invaders. He would pursue this path for the remainder of his illustrious career. However, Koch, perhaps due to his training as a physician and his experiences caring for the wounded in the Franco-Prussian War in 1870, took a more utilitarian approach towards the new science of microbiology. He was a practical man who believed that connecting specific bacteria to certain diseases would permit the rational use of hygiene to prevent these infections. Thus, his work became heavily focused on the development of laboratory methods to isolate bacteria in pure culture and on staining techniques with which to better visualize the organisms.

The dividends of Koch's approach rapidly accrued to the fledgling field of microbiology. One of his disciples, Paul Ehrlich, who would later be recognized as a cofounder of the field of immunology and would figure prominently in our story, devoted much of his early career in Koch's lab to developing the fundamental tenets of the technical aspects of staining bacteria so that microorganisms could be viewed under the microscope and differentiated from surrounding tissues and inflammation.[2] Ehrlich's work with methylene blue dye facilitated the visualization of bacilli in the lesions of tuberculosis, eventually leading Koch to prove, in 1882, a bacterial etiology of this great killer of the time. Christian Gram, a Danish physician also working in Berlin in the 1880s, extended Ehrlich's methods to demonstrate that adding an iodine solution to the violet dye and then exposing the sample to alcohol could differentially stain types of bacteria. This became the basis for the Gram stain, still widely used today in hospital laboratories to distinguish among categories of bacteria.

Koch, meanwhile, relentlessly pursued the idea of obtaining pure growth of a single bacterial type in artificial culture media.[2] The importance of this lay in its necessity in proving causality; the definitive proof that a specific microbe was the cause of a specific disease would require the isolation of the germ in pure culture from affected specimens of an individual or animal suffering from said malady. Although he initially recovered pure cultures of anthrax bacteria by injecting the organism into the blood of mice and then successively transferring the infected blood from mouse to mouse—a phenomenon known as "serial passage" and now understood to be related to the genetic selection of favored bacteria, analogous to Darwin's notion of natural selection—Koch was convinced that a technique was needed for the pure culture of bacteria using artificial substances—in vitro—that was therefore less labor intensive and less expensive.

Building upon a series of trial-and-error experiments, Koch soon devised a method for growing pure cultures of bacteria on a nutrient-fortified, gelatin base. He demonstrated the success of this technique at the International Medical Congress in London in 1881, attended by the most prominent men in the field—Lister and

Pasteur among them—and instantly became a celebrity scientist.[2] Koch's "plating technique" underwent a few minor modifications early on. First, the gelatin, which tended to melt at the temperature of the human body that bacteria tend to favor, was replaced with a different solidifying agent—agar—an algae-derived substance that was well known at the time in culinary circles for its use in jam-making and was suggested by the wife of one of his co-workers. Agar possessed the dual advantages of possessing a high melting point, thereby allowing it to remain solid at the 98.6°F body temperatures and having the ability to retain its liquid form at temperatures that permit it to be comfortably poured into laboratory glassware before solidification.

Richard Petri, one of Koch's assistants, instituted another minor, albeit critical modification to the technique in 1887. Petri conceived of a transparent, covered dish apparatus into which the liquid agar was poured, thus allowing for the repeated visual examination of the cultures without risking contamination by airborne organisms. Koch's technique for culturing bacteria using agar in these novel "Petri" dishes represented one of the simplest yet most significant advances in the history of medicine. It provides a classic example of how a seemingly trivial adjustment can propel a field forward by revolutionizing the tools of its trade. The technique remains in daily use today in microbiology labs and hospitals throughout the world, a testament to its lasting legacy.

Now, armed with the laboratory tools needed to determine whether specific germs were associated with specific diseases and heeding the newly minted criteria set down by Koch in 1882 to ascribe a bacterial etiology to an illness, physicians and scientists of the late nineteenth century presided over an unparalleled period of prolific discovery in the arena of medical microbiology. Within a span of twenty-five years, the last quarter-century of the 1800s, the specific bacterial etiologies of a number of the most dreaded diseases of that epoch were elucidated.

The list of infectious diseases with newly assigned bacterial causes reads like a "Who's-Who" scroll of lethality. Beginning with Koch's groundbreaking work with anthrax in 1876, that period witnessed the confirmation of bacterial causes of tuberculosis—the "captain of all these men of death"—in 1882; cholera, the elusive pathogen that terrorized the world in recurring pandemics of the nineteenth century, in 1883; typhoid, a disease of significant military import, in 1884; diphtheria, the cruelest of the childhood diseases—killing its young victims by suffocation—also in 1884; lobar pneumonia due to the pneumococcus, the most common and deadly bacterial infection of century's end, in 1887; tetanus, the cause of lockjaw and battlefield-related deaths, in 1889; and in 1894, plague, the culprit of recurring, explosive pandemics—most notably the Black Death of the fourteenth century—that altered the geopolitical history of Europe.[3] Additionally, malaria, the cause of millions of deaths around the world, was proven to be of microbial origin—though not a bacterium but a protozoal parasite—in 1896.

The nineteenth century ended with another discovery that would herald the next great era of medical microbiology. Agricultural scientists working contemporaneously in the Netherlands and in Russia determined that a filterable agent—too small to be trapped by the common devices used to detain bacteria—was responsible for the economically devastating "mosaic disease" of tobacco plants. These previously unidentified filterable agents, soon to be known as viruses, were beyond visualization by the microscopes of the time; hence, they were "submicroscopic." Viruses would be shown—over the first quarter of the dawning twentieth century—to be causally linked to at least 65 diseases of animals and humans.[4] Their discovery would eventually usher in a new discipline within microbiology and stimulate the next great period of scientific breakthroughs.

However, back in the nineteenth century, the medical world was busy applying the newly acquired knowledge to their patients' illnesses. Amid the flurry of scientific activity surrounding the host of newly recognized bacterial causes of clinically important infectious diseases of humans in the latter part of the nineteenth century was the identification of a novel pathogen that caused a well described, highly lethal, yet lesser known syndrome—cerebrospinal meningitis. The disease was marked by the dramatic onset and progression of signs and symptoms related to inflammation of the central nervous system (CNS)—the brain—the "cerebrum"—and the spinal cord. It was unique enough to be clinically distinct from the myriad other acute illness syndromes that were recognized among physicians and their patients of the era.

In 1887, Anton Weichselbaum, an Austrian physician and Professor of Pathological Bacteriology at the University of Vienna, reported finding small, round-shaped bacteria under the microscope in stained specimens of pus found overlying brain tissue during the autopsies of six individuals who had succumbed to cerebrospinal meningitis.[5] While he may not have been the first to see such germs in cases of the disease, he was the first to systematically study it the way of Koch. He grew pure cultures of the organisms via the newly described methods of the German physician and inoculated them into a variety of animals, successfully reproducing the lesions of meningitis in the brains of dogs and fulfilling Koch's postulates of causality—the latter having already acquired the status of dogma in late nineteenth century, European scientific circles.

Weichselbaum named the organism "*diplococcus intracellularis meningitidis.*" Translated into lay terms, the moniker described the appearance of the bug. It tended to occur in pairs—hence "diplo"; demonstrated a rounded shape ("cocci" refers to their round shape as seen under the microscope, as opposed to "bacilli," which describes the rod shape of some other bacterial species, such as anthrax); and it was found mostly within the white blood cells—hence, "intracellularis"—of patients with meningitis. White blood cells are the infection-fighting foot soldiers of the human immune system that circulate in the blood and are sent in to sites of infection to try to contain the invader; they are the principal component of the creamy-white pus that is seen in a variety of infections. Weichselbaum's organism rapidly became known as the "meningococcus." The organism was decolorized by the Gram stain, the latter described just a few years earlier in Berlin. Hence, the bacterial agent that appeared to cause the syndrome of acute cerebrospinal meningitis was a Gram-negative, intracellular diplococcus.

As we have seen, it was not until microbiology came of age in the latter part of the nineteenth century that many of the most infamous infectious diseases of nature could be explained and understood. Many, like plague, smallpox, and tuberculosis, were well-recognized and feared clinical syndromes long before their actual causes were identified. For some illnesses, such as diphtheria and rabies, the symptoms and signs were sufficiently distinct that they left little doubt as to the culprit; in others, such as anthrax among livestock and plague among human communities, the appearance and dynamics of recurring outbreaks were stereotypical enough in their characteristics as to warrant their specific diagnostic imprint. Still other disease syndromes, influenza and measles among them, remained problematic for early physician observers because they were somewhat nonspecific in clinical appearance. Influenza, a common and contagious acute infection of the respiratory tract, was difficult to discern from other respiratory diseases on the basis of signs and symptoms. Measles was at times confused with smallpox or other communicable diseases associated with fever and rash.

The syndrome of cerebrospinal meningitis was relatively new as compared with these other diseases of antiquity. It appears to have initially been recognized as a distinct entity by Vieusseux, who published the first report of the disease in the scientific literature in 1805.[6] He described a relatively small outbreak of an unusually dramatic illness that occurred in Geneva in the winter of that year that was characterized by its sudden onset with fever, vomiting, severe headache, and profound neck stiffness. The illness preferentially affected children—who frequently had seizures in the acute phases—and young adults; cases in older individuals were rare. He also observed that many of those who died, 26 in all, tended to succumb rapidly—some within twelve hours; others lasted up to five days. Vieusseux and a pathologist colleague found a bloody, gelatinous exudate covering the surface of the brain and pus on the underside and back of the brain during the autopsy of a case. The rest of the body and its organs seemed unaffected by the disease process.

Shortly after the Geneva epidemic, another outbreak of a disease with similar clinical and pathological attributes was recognized in the United States. The authors who reported the outbreak, however, were unaware of Vieusseux's cases. In 1806, two physicians from Medfield, Massachusetts, a sleepy rural town about seventeen miles south of Boston, described "the history of a singular and very mortal disease" in eight children characterized by the sudden onset of "violent pain in the head and stomach, succeeded by cold chills, and followed by nausea and puking…the eyes have a wild vacant stare…the heat of the skin soon becomes much increased…livid spots, resembling purple spots which appear in the last stages of certain fevers, appear under the skin, on the face, neck, and extremities…" until the patient's level of consciousness deteriorated into deep coma and death, generally over the span of hours.[7]

In one of the Medfield cases, that of a 15-month-old, they described "a very violent pulsation" of the fontanel—the soft spot at the vertex of the baby's head where the various bones that comprise the plates of the skull eventually fuse together. It takes about 18–24 months for the gap between the flat bones of the skull to completely close. Until then, anything causing increased pressure in the brain, such as hemorrhage, the growth of a brain tumor, or the inflammation associated with cerebrospinal meningitis, could cause bulging of the fontanel.

Five children in the initial Medfield report underwent autopsies. The findings were remarkably similar to those observed in Geneva, with bloody exudate and pus found around the brain and its coverings. The children's other organs seemed healthy. Although the diseases were identical, it is unlikely that there was any relationship, aside from a temporal one, between the outbreaks in Geneva and Massachusetts. But in the decade after the Medfield outbreak, epidemics of meningitis started appearing throughout New England and New York; by the 1830s, the disease had spread throughout most of the United States and parts of Canada.[8]

Although it was first recognized as a distinct entity in the reports of 1805 and 1806, epidemic meningitis had probably existed earlier than that. Outbreaks of illnesses of similar ilk—notably presenting with prominent and severe head pain, neck muscle rigidity, and acute onset with high fatality rates had been mentioned in various European sources as far back as the sixteenth century. But by the nineteenth century, the state of science was catching up with careful clinical observation, making it possible to more accurately—microbiologically—investigate this 'new' disease.

The study of the brain and the spinal cord—the elements comprising the CNS—dates back to the ancients. However, neurology, the study of diseases of the nervous system, like other medical disciplines, did not truly originate until the rise of anatomists and their science during the Renaissance. It evolved in parallel with advances in microscopy in the eighteenth and nineteenth centuries. By the time that acute, epidemic meningitis was recognized as a distinct clinical entity with its own specific, discrete bacterial etiology, most of the anatomy and much of the physiology of the CNS had been elucidated.

The human CNS is organized into three levels, reflecting not only an anatomical delineation but also a hierarchy of function. At the highest level is the cerebral cortex—the main portions of the brain that lie directly under the flat bones of the skull, or "cranium." It is structurally divided into two hemispheres, left and right, each with four sections, or lobes, named after their overlying skull bones: frontal, parietal, temporal, and occipital. The cerebral cortex is the body's main storage facility for information related to movement, sensory perception, language, emotion, and memories of past experiences.

The frontal lobes control executive thought functions; their rear area controls motor, or movement, functions of the body. The parietal lobes, behind the frontal lobes on top of the head, are charged with integrating incoming sensory information from a variety of sources throughout the body and orchestrating appropriate responses, which may involve enlisting the body's nerves and muscles to perform a variety of functions, such as withdrawing the hand from a hot stove. The temporal lobes, located on the lower sides of the head just above the ears, are primarily responsible for the processing of auditory information. The occipital lobes, at the back of the brain, process visual signals that come through nerve pathways from the eyes.

The CNS structures appear almost like a walking stick with a large, bulbous handle. In this example, the shaft of the cane represents the spinal cord; the handle represents the brain. Connecting the cerebral cortex portion of the brain—the handle of the cane—to the spinal cord is the subcortical region. This part of the brain, a dense collection of nervous tissue and nerve bundles, is divided into multiple, functionally distinct sections, comprising significantly less surface area than the cerebral cortex but of no less importance. It is primarily responsible for the control of life-sustaining, subconscious activities of the body such as breathing, heart rate, blood pressure, body temperature, and level of consciousness.

The subcortical part of the brain tapers seamlessly to form the spinal cord, a tightly wrapped collection of nerve tracts that runs—like thick electrical cables—up and down the length of the back. The spinal cord is held in place by the vertebrae—the triangular-shaped backbones—and it travels within the rings formed by the vertebrae, much like a shower curtain rod runs within the rings of the curtain. The long nerves within the cord branch at numerous points throughout their path into peripheral nerves that radiate towards all of the internal and external structures of the body like tapering tree branches; they carry sensory information from various internal and external body parts back to the brain and simultaneously relay motor or movement information from the brain out to the periphery. Not surprisingly, these long nerve branches are part of the peripheral nervous system, which along with the CNS, comprise the entire nervous system of vertebrate animals.

All of the structures of the CNS lie enclosed within three layers of coverings, collectively called the "meninges." The outer-most one, the dura mater, is a relatively thick, dense membrane that surrounds and protects the major blood vessels that nourish the tissues of the CNS. Beneath the dura lies the arachnoid mater, a thin film named for its spider web-like appearance that forms a loose-fitting sac to cushion the CNS. Finally, under the arachnoid is the pia mater, the most delicate of the membranes and the one that adheres directly to the surface of the brain and cord. The thin space between the layers of the arachnoid and pia—the subarachnoid space—contains cerebrospinal fluid (CSF), a normally clear body fluid that surrounds, bathes, and protects the brain and is continuously regenerated and recirculated within the CNS.

The term "meningitis" and the name of the causative agent of the epidemic form of disease—the meningococcus—derive from the involvement of the meninges by the organism's infectious process. In epidemic cerebrospinal meningitis, as demonstrated initially in the autopsy reports from Geneva and Medfield and confirmed subsequently over many years, bacterial infection spreads within the subarachnoid space, causing purulent exudate—pus—to accumulate along the surface of the brain. The CSF within that space is infected early in the process.

In the early years after the recognition of epidemic meningitis as a distinct clinical entity, it came to be known for a time as "spotted fever," due to the dramatic, albeit infrequent occurrence of pinhead or pea-sized purplish spots on the skin of the extremities, especially over clothing pressure points such as the waist and upper extremities. Because these spots were felt to be part of the clinical picture yet were in actuality only seen in a subset of cases, it was difficult to discern the actual numbers of cases of the disease. Additionally, because physicians of the time lacked the diagnostic tools of later generations, they depended on their astute physical examination skills and powers of observation to clinically differentiate epidemic meningitis from other "spotted fevers," especially the more common and less rapidly fatal typhus.[9, 10]

In the immediate aftermath of the Medfield outbreak, similar cases of meningitis were described from various towns and villages in Connecticut, upstate New York, Maine, and elsewhere in Massachusetts. In 1811, Elisha North of Connecticut, a general practitioner although without a medical degree at the time,[11] published a collection of the known medical experiences with epidemic meningitis in New England over the five years since it had first been described in the United States. In this collection are independent, anecdotal reports from experienced physicians who describe their initial encounters with this new disease.[12] The clinical descriptions they provide are all remarkably similar; most notable is the consistent way the disease course progressed in many of their patients—rapidly and inexorably to death.

Even in its early incarnations the disease, as we shall see and explain later, had a special predilection for military recruits. But unlike dysentery, malaria, tetanus, and other maladies of the field, cerebrospinal meningitis was largely a disease of troops billeted in barracks. Beginning with the American war with England in 1812, meningitis was noted to accompany recruits in this environment and was well described among troops embarked throughout the United States in the nineteenth century as well as garrisons throughout countries of Western Europe. Widespread occurrence of small outbreaks accompanied both the Union and Confederate armies during the U.S. Civil War. Although the number of cases paled in comparison to the millions of cases of diarrhea and dysentery that plagued troops in this conflict, the case mortality—those who died from the disease—was exceedingly high, rivaling only yellow fever in this regard.[13]

According to a comprehensive report issued in monograph form by an expert group convened by the Massachusetts State Board of Health to study the disease at the end of the nineteenth century, the footprints of epidemic meningitis to that point—known in some circles by its pseudonyms of "spotted" or "malignant spotted fever"—could be tracked via numerous focal outbreaks throughout the United States and more confined occurrences in Europe in the early part of the century to more widespread epidemics in the Western world. Despite relatively low absolute numbers of cases in comparison with other well-known diseases of the time such as cholera and smallpox, meningitis was associated with very high death rates, exceeding thirty percent in most reports. In Massachusetts alone, meningitis accounted for nearly 3,000 deaths in the last quarter of the nineteenth century.[14] By the latter part of the century, the disease had gone truly global, permeating parts of Asia, South America, and Africa.[14]

The patterns of early cerebrospinal meningitis epidemics differed in at least one important feature from those of other, more established infectious diseases. Classic epidemic diseases generally spread within households, whether related to a common environmental source, such as contaminated food or water, or from person-to-person transmission. Early meningococcal outbreaks, on the other hand, appeared as isolated events in areas that had hitherto been free of disease, and it was common to observe households with only one affected person. This character of meningitis epidemics would change as the nineteenth century progressed, in large part due to social changes that altered the population and the burgeoning association of epidemics with military settings, schools, urban areas, and other densely populated environments. The explanation for these observations would be discovered in due time, but this aspect led to early disagreement on whether cerebrospinal meningitis truly represented a contagious disease.

By the latter part of the nineteenth century, the entity of epidemic meningitis had become well recognized in medicine. The clinical presentation—signs and symptoms—had been well described. The course of disease had been well documented. The disease had been observed in most parts of the world; its outbreak characteristics—what would become known as the discipline of "epidemiology" based on the mid-century work of John Snow and others who used investigative techniques and statistics to describe epidemic disease patterns—were beginning to be understood. And before century's end, Weichselbaum had identified the germ that caused epidemic meningitis; the organism—the meningococcus—would be proven to satisfy Koch's supreme criteria for causality.

Amid the flurry of microbiologic activity in the final quarter of the century was another discovery that provides a final footnote to the early history of epidemic meningitis. Just a few years before Weichselbaum found the bacterial agent responsible for the disease, Albert Neisser, a German physician and contemporary of Koch, had discovered another diplococcus bacteria, this one in stained smears of pus recovered from the genital tract of patients with sexually transmitted diseases. He succeeded in growing the organisms—found to be the cause of the sexually transmitted disease gonorrhea—in pure culture. Although the disease had been known for centuries, the bacteria proved to be a novel type, and the genus—the first of two names generally used to categorize bacteria based on their degree of relatedness—was therefore named in Neisser's honor, as was customary at the time.[15]

Neisseria gonorrheae remains one of two species (the latter refers to the second name used to categorize and subgroup bacteria) of *Neisseria* known to commonly cause human disease, although other species of *Neisseria* have been identified as benign bacteria that normally may live as harmless "colonizers" in human throats. The other, disease-causing one is *Neisseria meningitidis*—the meningococcus—the cause of epidemic meningitis and subject of this book. Although the two germs cause markedly dissimilar clinical syndromes, they are closely related biochemically, as was learned early in their history and explains why they are grouped together. Additionally, molecular technology of the twentieth century has demonstrated that they are also closely related genetically, sharing more than ninety five percent of their genes. Despite this, the gonococcus generally causes a sexually transmitted disease—with some exceptions, including joint and bloodstream infections—while the meningococcus causes cerebral meningitis, albeit also with some exceptions.[16] Could the latter bug have derived from a mutation of the former that caused it to change the way it enters and attacks humans? Although we can still only speculate about its ancestral lineage, by the early twentieth century we had developed a solid understanding of the meningococcus and the deadly disease it causes in humans.

Chapter 4
A Very Mortal Disease

Each year millions of Muslims make their way to Mecca, the birthplace of Islam's prophet Muhammad and site of its holiest city, about 50 miles from the Red Sea on the western border of Saudi Arabia. This *Hajj*, the ritual pilgrimage to Mecca, is a conditional obligation to be performed at least once in the lifetime of every follower of Islam.[1] Early in its history, pilgrims arrived solely by sea or via caravan along numerous distinct overland routes from 'distant' lands like Syria, Iraq, and Egypt. In modern times, the sojourner is more apt to arrive by airplane from any number of places around the world.

Participants in the holy pilgrimage have at times been exposed to more than just prayer and reflection; infectious diseases have been constant companions of the worshippers throughout history. Epidemic diseases tend to thrive under environmental conditions that promote their spread from person to person, such as those engendered by large crowds that place people in close proximity to each other. Although this dynamic is amplified by indoor crowding—an explanation for the rapid spread of respiratory infections in schools, military barracks, and college dormitories—the overarching principle has to do with the density of people and the relative distances from one person's nose to that of another. The way most respiratory pathogens are spread from person to person is by tiny liquid droplets that get expelled from infected people through coughing, sneezing, or even breathing and then get inhaled by others in close—usually less than six feet—proximity.

Situations that bring together crowds of people with varying levels of health, especially those people who might harbor infectious agents or who might be vulnerable to them because of other medical conditions, have the potential to promote the spread of epidemic disease. Because the Hajj amasses immense groups of people from varying backgrounds together in close quarters and at least in earlier times under suboptimal sanitary conditions, it is not entirely surprising that serious health issues have accompanied this event.

A.W. Artenstein, *In the Blink of an Eye: The Deadly Story of Epidemic Meningitis*, DOI 10.1007/978-1-4614-4845-7_4, © Springer Science+Business Media New York 2013

In the nineteenth century, during the height of epidemic cholera throughout the world, it was this disease that was imported into Mecca, killing tens of thousands of pilgrims in its episodic occurrence between 1865 and 1912.[1] Cholera at the Hajj was eventually brought under control through the appropriate use of quarantine—the temporary isolation of non-ill individuals to ensure that they were not harboring a communicable disease—and the natural waxing and waning cycles of the infection worldwide. Seventy-five years later another epidemic disease—meningococcal meningitis—would become a major health threat to the masses on their spiritual journey, causing travel restrictions, policy changes, and sparking new outbreaks as pilgrims returned to their home soil carrying their infectious guest in their nasal passages.[2]

Most infections are initially recognized as distinct entities by the circumstances surrounding individual—"sporadic"—and epidemic cases and the clinical manifestations of their disease. The distribution, patterns, and determinants of infections are known as the epidemiology of disease; clinical manifestations refer to the symptoms—what the patient complains of—and signs—what the health care provider finds on examination—that the disease provokes.

Some illnesses, like the common cold, are recognized as syndromes. Colds can be caused by a variety of different respiratory viruses that share certain epidemiologic features and clinical manifestations. Epidemiologically, colds tend to occur in cooler months, affect younger individuals more frequently than older ones, and usually cause relatively mild illness. Clinically, colds are widely recognized by their symptoms: runny and/or stuffy nose, general malaise or feeling rundown, sore throat, cough, and in some cases fever. Most cases improve and resolve over a few days. It is difficult, based upon epidemiologic and clinical features alone to discern one cause of a cold from another. However, other infectious diseases, such as measles, influenza, or malaria, can be defined as specific entities by their distinctive clinical appearance in the context of certain epidemiologic patterns. Cerebrospinal meningitis falls into this category.

Sporadic—episodic—cases of bacterial meningitis can be caused by a variety of microorganisms, but more than nighty percent of cases in children and adults are caused by one of three bacteria: *Streptococcus pneumoniae*, the "pneumococcus"; *Neisseria meningitidis*, the "meningococcus"; and *Hemophilus influenzae*, H. flu.[3] Of these, the pneumococcus, so named because of its historical primacy in causing bacterial pneumonia—an acute infection of the lungs—accounts for the vast majority of adult cases of meningitis and more than a third of childhood cases. *Hemophilus influenzae*, originally but erroneously thought to be the cause of influenza at the turn of the twentieth century (an illness subsequently found to be caused by a virus in the 1930s), had played a dominant role in childhood bacterial meningitis until the introduction of effective vaccines three decades ago. It now accounts for only a small fraction of cases in developed countries.

Meningococcal meningitis accounts for approximately fifteen to forty percent of bacterial meningitis cases among children and young adults in the United States and is associated with a very high mortality rate—ten percent. Although the incidence of disease appears to have decreased somewhat in the United States over the past decade, for unclear reasons but perhaps in part related to vaccination,[3] meningococcal meningitis remains a significant cause of lethal, sporadic disease among children and young adults and occasional outbreaks in the same age groups. When epidemics do occur, they are usually confined to semi-enclosed, densely populated environments, such as college dormitories, prisons, military barracks, and child-care centers.

In the developing world, the dynamics of invasive, meningococcal disease are markedly different. There, meningococcal meningitis remains a global health problem of immense proportions. Outbreaks have occurred worldwide, from Brazil to China to New Zealand to Africa to the Hajj pilgrimage in Saudi Arabia. Children, adolescents, and young adults are primarily affected and are the unfortunate recipients of the death and nervous system destruction left in the wake of meningococcal epidemics.

The northern portion of sub-Saharan Africa is a region of tropical savannah that is characterized by two main seasons: a rainy season from June to September, and the dry season, which lasts from December to June and is punctuated by the "harmattan," a hot, dry wind that blows south from the Sahara desert, carrying sand and other particulate matter with it. Nearly 50 years ago, Leon Lapeyssonnie, a renowned French epidemiologist with substantial field experience in Africa, produced the definitive epidemiologic descriptions of the epicenter of worldwide epidemic meningitis.[4]

Lapeyssonnie's first assignment to Francophone Africa in 1942 involved a military investigation into the incidence and prevalence of trypanosomiasis — sleeping sickness, a disease causing widespread illness and death in French West African colonies in Bobo-Dioulasso, Upper Volta — now Burkina Faso. While there, he and his colleagues also witnessed firsthand the human toll of epidemic meningitis, which by that time was already a well-known cause of recurrent, explosive outbreaks in Africa.

Two decades later, after serving in a variety of leadership positions and achieving senior academic rank within the French public health system, Lapeyssonnie returned to Africa as a World Health Organization consultant to countries experiencing meningitis epidemics. Because of his stature in the field, he had access to the many official and unofficial reports that had been published over the preceding 30 years; he used these and his own astute observations to accurately define the epidemiology of meningitis in Africa. He comprehensively described this in the 1963 classic monograph that for the first time, referred to the affected area as the "African meningitis belt".[4]

Lapeyssonnie described the wave-like dynamics of epidemic meningitis in Upper Volta, Niger, Chad, Nigeria, and Sudan and underscored some of the characteristics that have continued to make the disease such a formidable public health problem, such as the impossibility of accurately predicting where or when epidemics will strike. He provided detailed descriptions of the focality, seasonality, and the kinetics of epidemics there. Additionally, he delineated the basic epidemiology and bacteriology of meningococcal epidemics in Africa: the overwhelming predominance of one type of germ — group A *Neisseria meningitidis* as the causative agent; the distribution of epidemics over two to three consecutive years; the age distribution of cases with a predominance in young children and teenagers; and the human costs engendered by the long-term, neurologic sequelae in those 'lucky' enough to survive an episode of meningitis—deafness, mental retardation, seizures, and amputation, due to compromise of the blood supply to limbs.[4]

The meningitis belt extends from Senegal in West Africa to western Ethiopia in the eastern part of the continent. Annual outbreaks there peak towards the end of the dry season and abruptly end with the onset of the rainy season. They tend to recur in cyclic fashion since they were first described in modern-day Nigeria in the early part of the twentieth century.[5, 6] Although the origin of meningococcal disease in West Africa is unclear, it may have arrived via holy pilgrims or by Arab traders or soldiers following pilgrim routes.[5]

Rates of disease in the African meningitis belt are significantly higher than those in developed countries, yet reported mortality—death—rates are similar—approximately ten percent. However, it is likely that an unknown number of deaths occur in remote areas of sub-Saharan Africa and are thus unreported and uncounted. Although outbreaks in this part of the world occur annually, larger epidemics recur every seven to twelve years. Just based on the sheer volume of cases in Africa, dozens to hundreds of thousands of deaths—as opposed to the dozens to hundreds of deaths in industrialized countries—occur there annually. More than 150,000 cases of meningococcal meningitis were reported in 1996—the largest African outbreak on record.[7]

Like its epidemiologic patterns, the clinical characteristics of meningococcal meningitis have become well established since its initial descriptions 200 years ago. But before a microbe such as the meningococcus can cause symptoms and signs, it must first infect its only natural host—humans. With any infection caused by any germ, there must always be an initial interaction between host—the patient—and pathogen—the germ. This first encounter can occur in a variety of ways. Infectious agents can be introduced to the host exogenously via the transfer of blood, such as might occur with a needlestick or a blood transfusion; by an insect bite as with malaria or Lyme disease; or by transfer from person to person by contact of an uninfected individual with contagious material from an infected one. Depending on the type of pathogen, the contagious material is typically carried on the skin or in the stool, or it is transmitted by secretions from the respiratory tract via a cough, sneeze, or simply during the act of breathing.

In some instances, the infecting germ does not need to be introduced to the host because it already resides there. It is well known that humans acquire a resident bacterial population—the "microflora"—very early in their post-fetal lives, coincident with their first breath and first meal. These bacteria are "colonizers"—members of the bacterial population that normally resides in relative harmony with most living things. They are found on the surface lining of most organs of the body; their relative burdens, however, are organ specific, with the skin—the largest human organ by surface area, large intestine, and vagina taking the prizes for the highest concentrations of normal bacterial inhabitants. In some cases, the normal bacterial flora are helpful to the humans they colonize, such as the important role they play in the production of certain forms of vitamin K in the intestines, or in their ability to populate valuable host turf, thus preventing other, more dangerous bacteria from setting up shop there. In other circumstances, they may provide little benefit to their hosts but are at least not harmful.

Humans and their resident bacteria usually live together symbiotically unless something happens to alter their relationship. A breach in the integrity of the bowel wall, such as may occur during surgery, allows some of its usual resident bacteria to gain entrance to the abdominal cavity or bloodstream, tissues and organs to which they are normally inaccessible. This may result in a life-threatening infection—peritonitis—caused by these usually cooperative germs. In other circumstances, such as occurs in critically ill patients in the intensive care unit, nonresident, dangerous bacteria present in the hospital environment can become colonizers, overtaking the usual, protective bacterial flora and setting the stage for life-threatening infections.

Neisseria meningitidis arrives in a potential host through the respiratory tract secretions of another person. Although not a typical member of the resident flora, it can behave as such—at least temporarily—colonizing the upper airways of humans. Then, after weeks to months in that role, it is either cleared out as the host develops an effective immune response to its presence, or in certain instances, it can become a malicious intruder, producing serious illness.

Therefore, despite its frequent, dramatic clinical presentation as a rapidly progressive infection of the central nervous system, the actual process of meningococcal infection begins in the upper respiratory tract, in the anatomical area where the nasal passages communicate with the back of the throat—the "nasopharynx." Once the bacterium gains entry into the nasopharynx from the environment, usually arriving via the cough, sneeze, or breathing of another person harboring the organism in their own nasopharynx less than six feet away, it is able to attach to cells on the surfaces of the upper airways. It accomplishes this feat by using a specialized docking-type of apparatus—its adhesive, antenna-like pilus—and several specific bacterial proteins that target markers on the surface of host cells. This interaction allows the organism to establish residence and multiply in the upper airways. At this point, the meningococcal journey can take one of two paths: it can either reside temporarily in the throats of healthy hosts—which is its usual path—or in a minority of individuals, it can gain access to the bloodstream and from there to the central nervous system, resulting in invasive meningococcal meningitis.[8]

Up to twenty-five percent of healthy adults transiently carry the meningococcus in their nasopharynx. Carriage is more common in adolescents and young adults than in children, but it is affected by a number of variables other than age. Carriage is facilitated by intimate contact occurring in crowded conditions and by damage to the upper respiratory tract induced by such things as smoking, viral infections, or perhaps trauma due to environmental conditions, such as that which may occur when the dry, hot, dusty Saharan harmattan fills the air and throats with irritants. In epidemic conditions, carriage rates may be increased, and thus human hosts may acquire the organism and spread it more rapidly. Because most carriage organisms are not the same strains that cause disease, carriers are usually asymptomatic. In fact, most will develop an immune response to the organism residing in their throats, that protects them against invasive disease by other, related but potentially dangerous strains of meningococcus.[9]

Certain situations, such as those found in military barracks or other environments that gather young, immunologically vulnerable individuals together for prolonged periods under crowded, intimate living conditions, favor the particularly rapid spread of the organism from nasopharynx to nasopharynx. This will either result in immunity to infection, or in the minority of cases, symptomatic disease. In those unfortunate individuals who develop invasive meningococcal disease, it is because the meningococcus does not persist in a symbiotic relationship with the host but instead behaves as an invader, penetrating the surfaces of cells in the nasopharynx and thus readily gaining access to the bloodstream.

What determines whether the meningococcus is a transient, well-behaved visitor that is subsequently removed by the development of an effective immune response or becomes a cause of serious, life-threatening meningitis? The answer appears to be determined by properties of both the organism and of the human host it inhabits.

Certain strains of *N. meningitidis* are potentially more dangerous than others. Those that have special "capsules" — structures made up of complex sugar molecules strung together to form a type of shield — are protected against the host's immune defenses, like a stealth bomber is protected from radar. Other features intrinsic to certain types of meningococci, such as factors that allow them to derive nutrition from their host or better penetrate host cells, make them more likely to invade into the bloodstream and find their way to the central nervous system.

In some cases, it is certain features of the human host that place them at higher risk of developing meningitis once the meningococcal bacteria enter their nasopharynx. People with specific flaws in their immune systems or those who have had their spleens removed may be unable to contain and fight the organism when it gets into their throats; some of these individuals may even suffer multiple, recurrent episodes of meningococcal meningitis. But most of the time, whether the human host or the bacteria gain the upper hand in their struggle for dominance is a matter of luck and timing.

The perturbations in body physiology caused by a disease state — its "pathophysiology" — represent the cumulative changes in the functional activity of different human cells, tissues, and organs engendered by a medical insult or injury to the body — one that is caused by cancer, infections, drugs, toxins, or others. This roadmap of functional disturbances in the human body is what actually results in the disease state that is commonly recognized by its clinical manifestations. Functional changes induced in certain types of cells lead to a chain reaction of events in other cells and tissues — all mediated by chemical signals.

These chemical-fueled, cellular reactions lead to further reactions that become amplified as more cells and tissues become involved, not unlike the way one domino falling affects the next ones down the line and in turn, causes multiple different branches of dominoes to fall. Various pathophysiologic processes may manifest themselves as distinct sets of symptoms and signs of illness; this explains why some diseases are quite characteristic in their appearance. However, because the repertoire of responses of the body's cells and tissues to various injuries is finite, some distinct disease entities share a common set of clinical presentations.

In many pathophysiologic states, it is the human immune system—not the triggering medical event—that causes much of the damage that we recognize as clinical disease. The immune system is a complex, highly organized cellular army that serves as the body's main line of defense against a variety of foreign invaders; it joins the battle by releasing an arsenal of chemical weapons—arms that sometimes lead to significant collateral damage. It is therefore helpful to think about many diseases as the combination of an initial insult—trauma, cancer, an autoimmune process, or an infection—and the subsequent way in which the body responds to it.[10]

The body's response to a triggering event is influenced by many factors. An individual's genetic background—the actual way their DNA lines up to form different genes within their cells—has a significant say in how their tissues and organs respond to changed circumstances. Similarly, a wide array of environmental and behavioral factors affects the pathophysiology of disease and therefore its clinical appearance. Exogenous factors like tobacco smoke, injection drug use, alcohol, crowded conditions, and poor hygiene may greatly affect the disease process. Endogenous factors, such as a person's anatomical features or the underlying function of their immune defense system, may also have a significant impact on the way diseases become manifest. Yet, another important determinant of pathophysiology and the clinical presentation of a disease process is the presence of other medical conditions—"comorbidities"—that contribute to the overall health of the person and dictate to some extent the way their tissues and organs behave in response to a new disease event.

With infectious diseases, all of the aforementioned elements may conspire to cause the clinically recognized, full-blown picture of disease. But since the inciting event is an invasion of the person—now the "host"—by a foreign substance—a germ, the body's natural tendency is to mount a highly aggressive counterattack in an attempt to expel the microbe, calling on the full capabilities of its immune system to lead the charge. Just as broken eggs are the innocent victims of making an omelet, the body's own cells and tissues may be victims of the onslaught unleashed by the well-intentioned immune system in response to bacterial invasion. This 'dual sword' is a survival tactic that in many instances causes the worst parts of the disease— all in an attempt to salvage the host.[10] Such is the case with meningococcal meningitis.

As we have seen, the immune response usually recognizes and removes meningococci that are temporarily colonizing the nasal passages. In those instances in which the germs are not cleared by an effective response, they may penetrate through cells on the surface of the nasopharynx and in so doing gain entrance to the bloodstream. There, the meningococcal organisms release endotoxin—a powerful, chemical complex produced by a variety of different bacteria. But endotoxin is not like other bacterial toxins that kill cells or change their function; instead, it is recognized by the human immune system as a foreign substance. This sets off an alarm signal to the defense forces that a microbial invader is in their midst—inducing a swift and exuberant inflammatory reaction in the host. This entire reaction cascade is actually the result of a vigorous release of chemical mediators of inflammation that serves to amplify and extend the pathophysiologic effects that were initiated by the meningococcal bacteria gaining entrance to the host's bloodstream—the domino effect again.

From the bloodstream, the germ crosses into the central nervous system by breaching the "blood–brain barrier," usually the staunchest and last line of defense in that highly protected compartment. The barrier is actually more virtual than real and comprises the tightly connected cells that lie beneath the blood vessels. Under normal physiologic conditions, this barrier stands guard over the central nervous system, protecting it from foreign substances. Although some of these may be unwanted, like germs, others may offer benefits to the host—such as medications; the barrier makes it difficult for all to pass through. However, in the setting of the vigorous inflammatory reaction incited by the presence of meningococci in the blood, the normally tight connections between the cells of the blood–brain barrier become loosened, allowing the bacteria to sneak through. Once inside the central nervous system, meningococci are free to create havoc; the inflammatory response they generate there is largely responsible for the clinical manifestations of meningitis.

The clinical manifestations of human disease—the signs, symptoms, and sequelae that alert a person—now a patient—and their health care providers that something in the body is terribly amiss, are not necessarily, therefore, simply due to the initial inciting event. Although the abnormally rapid and disordered growth of a certain cell type that is cancer, the inability to regulate the critical level of the body's sugar fuels that defines diabetes, and the unrestrained attack of the body's defense mechanisms against its own tissues in the case of lupus are all triggered by an insult—in many instances unknown—that changes bodily function, the clinical clues to disease often result from secondary effects. In meningococcal meningitis, the bacteria cause symptoms and signs indirectly through their release of endotoxin and their entrance into the central nervous system—both accompanied by a massive activation of the body's immune and inflammatory response—causing many of the clinical findings.

The symptoms and signs of meningococcal meningitis had been fairly consistently described in the various case reports and series that began with the publications from Geneva and Medfield in 1805 and 1806, respectively, and continued through the published reports of outbreaks in the United States, Canada, and Europe during the nineteenth century. Sir William Osler of Johns Hopkins, perhaps the most accomplished physician of early twentieth century America and author of the first, comprehensive, modern Western textbook of medicine, provided an accurate and thorough summary of the clinical features—the signs and symptoms—of meningococcal meningitis in a turn-of-the-century lecture to physicians in London.[11] He described the acute onset of a severe headache, "without warning, while at work, or awakening from a sound sleep, comes the pain in the head"; an invariable fever that is unpredictable in its pattern; the common occurrence of various types of skin rashes, including lesions that looked like tiny blood spots—"petechiae"—on the limbs and trunk; and the extreme neck stiffness that accompanied cases of cerebrospinal meningitis. Several physical exam maneuvers that demonstrate the profound neck stiffness are eponymously named for physicians treating patients with meningitis in the late nineteenth century.

The sudden onset of fever, severe headache, and neck stiffness results from the spread of meningococci from the nasopharynx through the bloodstream with subsequent invasion of the central nervous system, causing inflammation that involves the coverings of the brain. Other symptoms or signs, such as nausea, vomiting, mental confusion, and sensitivity of the eyes to light—photophobia—may also frequently accompany meningococcal meningitis. Although this constellation of clinical findings is not specific for meningococcal disease and can be seen in some other forms of bacterial meningitis, the epidemiology—especially in its epidemic form— and its rapidly progressive course in individuals, is highly suggestive.

Although meningitis is the most common clinical manifestation of meningococcal disease, other forms of clinical illness may occur once the organism becomes invasive. These forms of disease may occur either with or without the involvement of the central nervous system. Frequently, meningococci can be found circulating in the bloodstream in patients with meningitis; fortunately, only a minority of these patients experiences an overwhelming systemic infection—meningococcal sepsis or "meningococcemia" (the "emia" syllable appended to medical terms connotes organisms circulating in the bloodstream; hence, "bacteremia" means bacteria in the blood and "viremia" means viruses in the blood)—that is almost uniformly fatal.

Meningococcemia is a highly deadly syndrome characterized by fever, a progressive rash—comprising a mixture of petechiae, bruising, and occasionally gangrene of the fingers or toes—and persistent, low blood pressures—shock. The severe shock seen with meningococcemia is a consequence of the massive inflammatory response that takes place in the blood vessels, leading to their collapse. A combination of persistent shock and ongoing, destructive inflammatory activity throughout the blood vessels of the body results in the failure of multiple organ systems— kidneys, lungs, and in some cases, the adrenal glands. Another consequence of the pathological release of chemical mediators of inflammation: blood coagulation mechanisms are dysregulated, leading to both hemorrhagic complications as well as the inappropriate formation of blood clots. The clots block blood flow to vital organs and the limbs, exacerbating organ failure and leading to tissue death—gangrene— of fingers, toes, or even entire arms or legs. Other clinical manifestations of meningococcal disease that may occur in the absence of meningitis include pneumonia and other respiratory tract infections, and infections of joints, the genitourinary system, the eyes, or the sac surrounding the heart.[12]

Although meningococcal meningitis as a clinical entity was well understood by the end of the nineteenth century, it remained a highly deadly disease, killing the majority of those affected. Treatment for the disease was still as it was in 1806: symptomatic, "alexipharmic"—antidote—therapy.[13] In those fortunate enough to survive a bout with the disease, many were left with significant disability, such as hearing loss, limb loss, or chronic cognitive deficits. Perhaps the most notorious feature of meningococcal meningitis—whether in its sporadic form or its epidemic form—was the young patient's extremely rapid descent from health to profound illness to death "in the blink of an eye."

Chapter 5
Early Approaches at Therapy

As the nineteenth century gave way to the twentieth, the dramatic revolution in microbiology engendered by the work of Pasteur, Koch, and their disciples began to translate into advances in medicine. In the United States, nowhere was this more evident than at Johns Hopkins in Baltimore, the home of Osler and other giants of early, modern medicine. The medical school there was founded in 1893 with William Welch as its inaugural dean, and it rapidly became the breeding ground for America's best-trained physicians. However, the burgeoning epicenter of medical research in the United States would be the newly created Rockefeller Institute, located on an isolated, windswept vista on the Upper East Side of Manhattan. There, the mysteries of disease would begin to be unraveled, leading to rapid advances in the therapeutic approach to many illnesses including a number of the most important bacterial infections of the time — meningococcal meningitis among them.

The national unification engendered by the conclusion of the Civil War allowed the extension of Northern industrialization to the rest of the country. For ambitious, industrious, self-made young men like Andrew Carnegie and John D. Rockefeller, it represented a fertile opportunity for advancement. Around the same time period that Koch proved a microbial etiology of tuberculosis and Pasteur demonstrated the efficacy of a rabies vaccine in humans, Rockefeller's company — Standard Oil — was refining more than ninety percent of America's oil.[1]

As Rockefeller's capitalistic success grew, so did his philanthropic activities. No doubt much of this part of his personality derived from his strict Baptist upbringing. He contributed generously to a variety of charitable causes, many of them aligned to priorities within the Church, including hospitals and public welfare projects. By the last decade of the nineteenth century, his annual contributions were worth hundreds of millions of dollars in today's currency value. He needed a deputy to manage just the philanthropic side of his business activities. In 1889, he would meet a cleric who would do just this — and help him change the course of medical history.

A.W. Artenstein, *In the Blink of an Eye: The Deadly Story of Epidemic Meningitis*,
DOI 10.1007/978-1-4614-4845-7_5, © Springer Science+Business Media New York 2013

Reverend Frederick T. Gates, executive secretary of the American Baptist Education Society, had risen meteorically from his upbringing in rural poverty through ministerial work in Minneapolis, to a position of statewide leadership among Minnesota Baptists. His success was a testament to both his personal attributes and his flair for fundraising. His appointment as essentially a development officer in the Baptist national Education Society placed him in the circles of some of the wealthiest men in the country. Perhaps the most prominent of these individuals—Rockefeller—was so impressed with Gates' financial and analytic prowess that he gave him stewardship over all of his non-Standard Oil related investments as well as his philanthropic activities.

By the end of the nineteenth century, Gates was working primarily with John D. Rockefeller, Jr. on the philanthropic side of the Rockefeller financial empire; Junior had joined the family business after graduating from Brown in 1897. That same year, according to Gates' own retrospective account of the origins of the concept of the Rockefeller Institute of Medical Research, the Reverend became aware of the vast deficiencies in medical science as compared with the natural sciences; he envisioned an institution in which physicians could investigate important scientific questions unencumbered by the demands of a clinical practice. Although he had observed the shortcomings in medical education while serving as a pastor tending to the sick and interacting with physicians during his tenure in Minneapolis in the 1880s, his personal epiphany regarding the many gaps in medical knowledge of the era apparently stemmed from a thorough reading of Osler's *Principles and Practice of Medicine*—most likely the second edition of this definitive text—while vacationing with his family in the Catskills.

Gates' boss was also inclined towards medical philanthropy. The senior Rockefeller had always taken an interest in medicine—homeopathic medicine—presumably borne from early childhood memories of his grandmother's herbal remedies prepared from a "physic bush" in their backyard in upstate New York.[2] Throughout his life, Rockefeller maintained an appreciation for homeopathic medicine and in fact, insisted that it be equitably represented in his philanthropic activities. This remained a chronic, simmering debate within the dynasty.[1]

As with many investments made by Rockefeller during his long, successful career, timing was critical, and the timing for medical philanthropy in turn-of-the-century America was ripe. In the two great medical science capitals of Europe—Paris and Berlin—research institutes had been established for their most prominent national figures in this arena—Pasteur and Koch, respectively. Private benefactors had built the Pasteur Institute; the Prussian government had supported the Koch Institute for Infectious Diseases.

In the United States, advances in medical science were closely allied with those in medical education. Practitioners for whom medicine was an occupation and teaching it was an uncompensated chore had stunted the development of medical education under a long tradition of on-the-job apprenticeship training of would-be physicians. This situation began to change in the latter part of the nineteenth century with reform and reorganization of some of the nation's oldest and most prestigious medical schools such as Harvard, Penn, and the University of Michigan—much of it facilitated by faculty members returning from scientific training in the venerable laboratories of France, England, and most notably, Germany.

The first and truest union of medical education and research with clinical medicine occurred with the opening of the medical school at Johns Hopkins University in 1893, a defining moment in the rise of modern American medicine. The hospital, founded by an 1873 bequest from Johns Hopkins, an entrepreneur who had made much of his substantial fortune with the Baltimore and Ohio Railroad, opened its doors in 1889 with such luminary Department Chairs as Welch in Pathology, Osler in Internal Medicine, and Halstead in Surgery.[3] Four years later Welch, himself trained in Koch's laboratory in Berlin, was the first Dean of the new medical school and had organized it into its preclinical departments, each with laboratories directed by trained scientific investigators and with full-time clinical faculty directing the hospital's clinical areas.[4]

Gates' vision of a research facility in which the best and brightest medical scientists could creatively explore the fundamental, scientific questions related to a broad range of diseases was analogous to the Hopkins model for medical education. To allow for the uninterrupted pursuit of medical research, investigators would work without concern for economic pressures—the faculty of the institute would be fully salaried—or teaching duties. Initially, the institute was organized without a university affiliation largely for this reason, although the decision was also influenced by the importance of avoiding a slight of homeopathic medicine. Rockefeller Sr. was, after all, a lifelong proponent of homeopathic medicine, and it was understood that the existing scientific medical universities were the purview of the elite, 'regular'—allopathic—physicians.[1]

Gates initially proposed the formation of an American institute, similar to the Pasteur Institute in Paris, in a memo to his boss in July 1897. As was Rockefeller's habit, probably gleaned from maternal lessons internalized at a young age, he tended to allow issues to "simmer" before returning a decision.[2] During this time, the ensuing four years, Gates and Junior performed their own due diligence towards their now shared goal; a consultant was hired to study and report on European models of such institutes, and medical experts were debriefed and encouraged to weigh in on the potential importance of such an undertaking to the advancement of medical science. The death of one of Rockefeller Senior's grandchildren in early 1901 of scarlet fever—a disease of unknown cause and for which there was no effective therapy at the time—tragically illustrated the need for the kind of research efforts proposed for the Institute. This event may have ultimately helped to crystallize Senior's decision to fund Gates' grand vision.

In June 1901, the Rockefeller Institute opened for business, largely as a grants organization in temporary quarters over its first few, formative years. Welch, then dean at Hopkins and widely considered the major force in American medical science of the era, was recruited to help organize the new Institute and to serve on its first Board of Directors. It was on his recommendation that his friend and colleague Simon Flexner, one of his former pathology trainees at Hopkins, was selected to the Board;

Flexner subsequently became the inaugural Director of the Institute's laboratories. By 1904, the laboratories within the Institute had begun their own research programs, generously supported by Rockefeller.[5]

Flexner was one of nine children of German-speaking Jewish parents reared in penury in Louisville, Kentucky.[6] Flexner's early life failed to presage his later accomplishments; he dropped out of school at the age of 14 and was directionless through his teenage years until a brush with death due to typhoid fever seemed to ignite a sense of intellectual purpose in him. After an apprenticeship with a local pharmacist, he clerked in his older brother's drugstore and there, through observing discussions of cases between physicians, became interested in medicine.

Because most medical education in the United States even in the late nineteenth century was still purely didactic and provided by local practitioners, Flexner arranged to attend a series of clinical lectures—at reduced fees due to his limited financial circumstances—and subsequently received a medical degree from the University of Louisville in 1889. In 1891, he began a fellowship in pathology and bacteriology, both new educational initiatives in select U.S. hospitals, under the tutelage of Welch, the Chair at the newly minted hospital at Johns Hopkins. When Hopkins opened its Medical School two years later, Flexner was given a faculty appointment in pathology.

After a brief stint as professor of pathology at the University of Pennsylvania from 1899 to 1901, during which he was appointed to the Board of Directors of the newly formed Rockefeller Institute for Medical Research, he accepted the offer to become the first director of the nascent Institute's laboratories, arriving there in 1902 and remaining in that position for 33 years, the last ten of which he spent directing the entire Institute's activities. Besides Simon, one other member of the Flexner family left a lasting legacy in the arena of academic medicine; younger brother Abraham's landmark study of medical education in the United States and Canada—the "Flexner report"—published in 1910. This report is credited with stimulating the first major reform in American medical education and creating the basis of the modern medical profession. Ironically, it also directly led to the end of the traditional, practitioner-driven medical degree programs—like the one that brother Simon had attended two decades earlier.

The early years at the Rockefeller Institute witnessed the development of a medical science research climate that rivaled that of the most prestigious of the European centers. Flexner, in his role as director, recruited a group of researchers who would become some of the most recognized names in their fields over the next few decades and who would make seminal discoveries that would lead to important medical advances. Eugene Opie, who as a medical student had been the first to observe that diabetes was associated with damage to specific cells in the pancreas, joined from Welch's lab at Johns Hopkins. Hideyo Noguchi, who initially conducted research on the deleterious effects of snake venom—housing boxes of live rattlesnakes in the lab—but would later demonstrate that syphilis caused progressive neurologic disease and who would die tragically of yellow fever while engaged in vaccine research in Africa, had known Flexner during his tenure at the University of Pennsylvania. Alexis Carrel, a French surgeon who would receive the Nobel Prize in 1912 for his work on tissue preservation, vascular grafting, and organ transplantation and whose research on tissue culture techniques would—almost half a century later—directly pave the way for vaccines against many of the most important viral diseases of humans, was brought to the Institute's laboratories from Europe.[5] At Rockefeller, scientists found a nurturing environment in which they could engage in—by today's standards—'high stakes' research with intellectual freedom and generous funding. Flexner was the common denominator; his vision for this type of work was imprinted on the Institute early on, and it permeated his own scientific efforts as well.

Even before his appointment as director of the new Rockefeller Institute laboratories, Simon Flexner was no stranger to the study of cerebrospinal meningitis. In 1892, as a 29-year-old pathology fellow at Hopkins, he had been sent to investigate an outbreak of the disease in the mining and manufacturing city of Cumberland, Maryland—in that state's western, Appalachian region.[7] Once in the newly minted laboratories at Rockefeller, it was not long before he was called upon again to lend his scientific prowess to the meningitis problem. However, now he had the benefit of applying 13 years of additional knowledge and technologic advances in the field of microbiology and, of course, he presided over state-of-the-art facilities in which to perform his investigations.

In the early 1900s, meningococcal epidemics were reported in several American, Canadian, and European cities. New York City was particularly hard hit in 1904–1905; over 4,000 cases accompanied by over 3,000 deaths from meningitis were recorded that season.[5, 8] In 1905, the Health Department of New York City appointed a commission to investigate the epidemic. As the director of the premier research institution in New York—the Rockefeller Institute's laboratories—Flexner was invited to become a member of the commission and to assist with the microbiologic studies. He quickly identified the causative organism as *Diplococcus intracellularis*—the meningococcus—known since Weichselbaum's work two decades earlier. His initial microbiologic studies confirmed that the meningococcus was a fragile organism that both lost its infectivity on subculture and was difficult to work with.[9] Always the careful scientist, Flexner insisted that all suspect cases of meningitis in New York undergo lumbar punctures—spinal taps—to allow for appropriate bacteriologic studies on the spinal fluid. This diagnostic test would figure prominently in his subsequent efforts at treating the disease.

Although the precise originator of the lumbar puncture technique for obtaining cerebrospinal fluid remains controversial, as priority has been variously ascribed to Heinrich Quincke, a German internist, American neurologist James Corning, and Walter Wynter, an English physician, the procedure was probably first applied—albeit using distinct techniques by different practitioners—in the period between 1885 and 1891.[10, 11] The procedure involved inserting a drainage apparatus—initially a type of rubber tube mounted on a solid trocar but subsequently on hollow needles—through the skin of the back into the space between the vertebral bones of the lower back. The needle was then advanced until the outermost layers that cover the spinal cord—the dura and arachnoid mater (the same outer coverings of the brain)—were punctured, marking the subarachnoid space. Once there, cerebrospinal fluid (CSF) drained through the needle and could be analyzed for various chemical and cellular constituents to make the diagnosis of meningitis.

As first performed, lumbar puncture—the term coined by Quincke—was used as a therapeutic procedure to remove CSF and thus potentially alleviate the disabling headaches in children suffering increased pressure in their brains related to either hydrocephalus—'water on the brain'—or tuberculous meningitis. Shortly thereafter, lumbar puncture began to be used for diagnostic purposes—to examine the CSF for evidence of inflammation or bacterial organisms—a circumstance for which it is still used today. Fourteen years later, Simon Flexner would introduce an additional use of the procedure.

Because Flexner's pathology training and his experiences at the university centers of Europe had taught him the importance of animal models—an investigative approach that he followed throughout his career, he furthered his studies of the biology of meningococcus through a series of bacterial challenge studies in rodents. He soon determined that mice and rats were resistant to large doses of the organisms when delivered by the intravenous route but intraperitoneal challenges—injections into the abdominal cavity—led to fatal infection in some young guinea pigs.

Flexner also performed a number of experiments using goat antiserum, a material which he derived from injecting goats with sublethal quantities of meningococcal bacteria—enough to stimulate their immune systems but not enough to kill them—and harvesting the serum fraction of their blood—the liquid portion without any of the blood cells—after the animal had mounted an effective immune response. The serum of these "immunized" animals contained antibodies—large proteins produced by immune cells in response to germs or other foreign substances in the bloodstream—and these molecules served to neutralize the invading bacteria. The activity of antibodies results from their capacity to essentially grab onto and sequester foreign invaders by a complex series of reactions that renders the germ unable to cause trouble. Flexner found that the antimeningococcal antiserum failed to prevent progression of infection if given subcutaneously but could reverse the fatal syndrome if given intraperitoneally and concurrently with the meningococcal challenges.[12]

The concept that serum derived from animals after their injection—immunization—with sublethal doses of bacterial organisms could have value as a therapy for infectious diseases had been pioneered by the work of Emil von Behring and Shibasaburo Kitasato working with the bacterial causes of diphtheria and tetanus in Koch's Institute of Infectious Diseases in Berlin about 15 years earlier. Diphtheria, one of the most dangerous infections of childhood through the early twentieth century, caused severe inflammation of the upper airways, making it a particularly cruel infection—killing its young victims by suffocation. Tetanus, known as "lockjaw" because of the characteristic and dramatic neuromuscular spasms of the jaw and neck muscles that it caused, was also a significant, albeit sporadic cause of mortality at the time. Tetanus was a particularly important cause of disease in combat settings because it tended to enter the body through traumatic wounds. In both cases, toxins produced by the bacteria were responsible for the pathophysiology of disease.

Behring and Kitasato showed that they could induce an "antitoxin" effect when they injected sera subcutaneously—under the skin—that had been harvested from animals challenged with nonlethal doses of either tetanus or diphtheria bacilli into other animals. This effect protected the recipient animals from death. Moreover, sera obtained from the protected animal could subsequently be used to convey immunity to a third animal—defining the concept of "passive transfer" of immunity. Behring performed such experiments in progressively larger animals, including sheep and horses, eventually winning the inaugural Nobel Prize in 1901 for the discovery of "serum therapy"—nearly a decade after his sheep-derived diphtheria antitoxin had made its way into clinical practice, its favorable effect on mortality confirmed in studies by Pasteur's protégé, Roux, in Paris children's hospitals.[13]

In the United States, William Park, director of the nation's first municipal infectious diseases diagnostic laboratory in New York City, advanced diphtheria antitoxin therapy into the realm of public health in the early days of the new century. His boss, Herman Biggs, a member of the original board of scientific directors of the Rockefeller Institute, had observed the production of diphtheria antitoxin while visiting Koch's Institute in 1894 and had been favorably impressed with the activity. Upon his return, he instructed Park to immediately develop a production plan for antitoxin.

Park's laboratory developed a strain of bacteria that yielded highly potent toxin, which was subsequently employed to raise effective antitoxin in horses—preferred serum sources because of their relatively large blood volume.[14] Park arranged for stocks of high potency horse antitoxin to be stored in drug stores throughout New York City, along with diagnostic throat-swab culture kits, so that physicians could have access to early diagnosis and treatment of patients with diphtheria. A similar model was later employed in other U.S. cities.

Flexner's involvement in the New York City meningitis outbreak of 1904–1905 occurred amidst the flurry of scientific activity and clinical enthusiasm for the use of diphtheria antitoxin that accompanied the last decade of the nineteenth and turn of the twentieth centuries. Always the careful scientist, he deemed it necessary to first develop a large animal model of meningococcal meningitis; he thus expanded his rodent studies using monkeys. After perfecting techniques in which he could reliably access cerebrospinal fluid—via lumbar puncture—in these nonhuman primates, he succeeded in creating a model of meningococcal meningitis by introducing the bacteria "intrathecally"—directly into the spinal canal and the cerebrospinal fluid compartment. The resultant infection mimicked what was seen in humans; stained smears of the spinal fluid showed polymorphonuclear leukocytes—infection-fighting white blood cells—as well as meningococci within and outside of these cells. The pathologic findings in the central nervous systems of these monkeys showed the presence of severe meningitis.[15]

Flexner thus began a series of critical experiments in July 1906 using antimeningococcal antiserum. At the time, he was fully aware of similar, contemporaneous work in Germany using guinea pigs and of a report using horse antimeningococcal antiserum inoculated directly into the spinal canal of humans with meningitis. The latter experiment, performed by German bacteriologist Georg Jochmann in 1905—although not yet published at the time of Flexner's work—clearly established Jochmann's priority for the concept. Jochmann had presented his results at a German medical conference in the spring of 1906.[5] However, Flexner performed rigorous scientific investigations to determine whether the intrathecal use of antiserum had validity in the treatment of meningococcal meningitis and therefore deserves credit for assessing the intervention in a systematic way.

Flexner hypothesized that because the pathologic lesions of the disease in both monkeys and humans began in the meninges and progressed to the brain and spinal cord, it may be important to deliver the therapy directly to the source of the problem. Using homologous antiserum—material derived from the same animal species in which it would be subsequently used for therapy—given concurrently with an intrathecal bacterial challenge or two to four hours after challenge, he demonstrated that the meningococcal infection appeared to be arrested in three animals.[16] A fourth monkey given antiserum after bacterial challenge died. Thus, three out of four animals given antiserum survived an otherwise lethal bacterial challenge, allowing Flexner to remark that the results were "sufficiently encouraging to be more widely and closely studied."

Despite the promising data, Flexner stopped short of extrapolating them to human disease and exercised special caution regarding the use of intrathecal injections in humans—arguing instead for further experiments in monkeys. However, realizing the importance of these observations and perhaps driven by the need to establish his own scientific priority, Flexner published his results in an August 1906 paper in the widely read *Journal of the American Medical Association*—a mere four weeks after the last monkey experiment—yet four months after Jochmann's presentation in Germany.[16]

A word about scientific priority is warranted. This concept was neither new in Flexner's time nor has it been relegated to obscurity since. In the realm of science, as in other disciplines involving innovation, it refers to the necessity of establishing a lineage of novel findings—"planting the flag"—so as to be recognized as the discoverer or originator of new information or "intellectual property," as it is now known. Often motivated by potential fame, fortune, or authority in the field, priority may serve medical science well; history has shown that competition between laboratories and investigators—like the race between Pasteur and Koch to find the cause of cholera, ultimately won by Koch—often leads to more rapid advances, as long as all participants follow the principles of ethics and fairness that must accompany such research. However, history is also replete with examples in which politics and personal animosities play a role in scientific priority and, as we shall see later, such issues became manifest in early meningococcal meningitis research.

In science, priority is generally established by the publication of results in scientific journals. With the rise of industrial science and biotechnology, the submission of patents has become a progressively more common route when priority involves new technical advances or products. Although Flexner's carefully planned and executed laboratory investigations represented important incremental advances in serum therapy for meningitis, the concept had clearly been informed by Jochmann's experiments using intrathecally introduced serum in 1905.[17] Nonetheless, the work coming from the Rockefeller Institute created momentum for the use of antimeningococcal antiserum therapy in humans as cases mounted during continuing U.S. outbreaks in the early twentieth century.

Despite Flexner's notes of caution in the conclusions of the initial paper describing his monkey studies, it was not long before an opportunity arose to use intrathecally delivered antiserum to treat humans with meningococcal meningitis. In 1907, epidemic disease struck Ohio. During the first quarter of the year, 18 cases of meningococcal meningitis were recorded around Castalia, a small rural village of 600 people near Lake Erie in the north-central part of the state; twelve of the eighteen patients died. Dr. L.W. Ladd, a Cleveland internist and a Johns Hopkins medical graduate, was aware of Flexner's animal studies and managed to obtain a supply of the horse antiserum from the Rockefeller Institute. He had treated the last three cases in the Castalia epidemic with intrathecal antiserum; all of the patients survived.[18] But because three of the Castalia cases recovered without the benefit of serum therapy, Flexner remained unconvinced of its therapeutic effect.

Not long after the Castalia outbreak and not far away, the city of Akron experienced epidemic meningitis. Intrathecal antiserum was used to treat 11 hospitalized cases at Akron City Hospital; eight of those treated survived, whereas eight of nine cases that were managed outside of the hospital without serum therapy ended fatally.[18] Ladd subsequently treated another thirty cases with antiserum in Cleveland in the spring of 1907; five of these died. Overall in these Ohio outbreaks, there were eight deaths among twenty-seven cases treated with antiserum, a fatality rate of thirty percent—as compared to a fatality rate of at least seventy-five percent in the untreated. Antiserum therapy performed even better in those who received it within seventy-two hours of symptoms—nighty percent survived. The results prompted the use of "Flexner's antiserum" in a series of other, nearly concurrent outbreaks in the United States in New York and Philadelphia, and in the United Kingdom, in Edinburgh, Scotland and Belfast, Ireland.

From 1907 to 1913, Flexner's horse antimeningococcal antiserum was probably used to treat thousands of patients around the world. It was distributed from the Rockefeller Institute to treating physicians at no cost with the caveat that data relating to the therapeutic use of the antiserum were to be sent back to Flexner. He subsequently summarized the results of nearly 1,300 treated patients in a series of publications that made a "forceful argument" that treatment with intrathecal antiserum—especially early in the course of disease—lowered the meningitis death rate from a baseline of seventy-five to eighty-five percent to approximately thirty percent.[19, 20]

Such a dramatic improvement in the outcome of this otherwise uniformly fatal infection with antiserum therapy brought public accolades to Flexner. It was probably the most important, personal scientific contribution of his career, although certainly his thirty three year tenure as Director at Rockefeller and the scores of contributions made by researchers that he personally recruited remain his lasting legacy in medical science. The Rockefeller Institute also received significant favorable publicity from its role in antiserum therapy for meningococcal meningitis. This proved to be a major stimulus to convince John D. Rockefeller to donate the new funds necessary for the construction of the Institute's Hospital—one that would be devoted solely to the care of medical research patients.

Not everyone in the field embraced the concept that the Rockefeller Institute deserved all of the public tributes it received regarding serum therapy. Park, the accomplished Director of the New York City Department of Health diagnostic laboratories and acknowledged expert on the subject of serum therapy, apparently bristled at the notion. When Flexner's Institute—not his Health Department laboratory—was incorrectly given credit for supplying antimeningococcal serum during an outbreak in Texas in 1912, Park raised the issue of scientific priority, publicly reminding people that it was Jochmann—not Flexner—who first developed the idea to use antiserum via an intrathecal route in patients.[14] Park was probably motivated both by personal ego as well as by political realities—still applicable today—that his laboratory's research funding was tied to some extent to the public perception that its contributions were important and continuous.

The final chapter in antimeningococcal serum therapy was written over the two decades that followed. Other public health institutions began producing their own horse antiserum, and a standard intrathecal administration kit was developed.[21] Serum therapy became the standard of care for meningococcal meningitis and continued as such until the late 1930s. During World War I mobilizations, serum therapy was used to manage outbreaks among troops.

Maxwell Finland, working in the Thorndike Laboratory at Boston City Hospital, applied a similar therapeutic approach in patients with pneumococcal pneumonia using type-specific pneumococcal antiserum.[22] He showed significant improvements in overall mortality among treated patients; as with meningococcal meningitis, these were especially striking in those treated with antiserum within three days of illness onset. Given the high prevalence and mortality of pneumococcal disease at the time—the 1920s and 1930s—this should have been a major therapeutic triumph. But events occurring in a German industrial laboratory during the same timeframe would forever change the therapeutic approach to infectious diseases.

Chapter 6
Antibiotics and Survival of the Fittest

"Flexner's serum" had a significant and dramatic impact on the uniformly poor prognosis associated with meningococcal meningitis in the early decades of the twentieth century, reducing the overall mortality by more than fifty percent and providing the first real glimmer of therapeutic hope in the century-long history of this disease. Similarly, serum therapy for pneumococcal disease — the most lethal of the common bacterial diseases of the time — showed substantial early promise during the 1920s and 1930s. It seemed at that juncture as if this would be the path towards managing some of the most dangerous bacterial infections of the era. However, an abrupt shift — a paradigm shift — was about to take place in medical science, one that would lead to a transformational change in the way in which infectious diseases were treated. In the late 1930s, this revolution would not only alter the prognosis of patients suffering from these maladies but would also alter the history of medical science — at least temporarily.

Throughout human history and until the latter portion of the nineteenth century, medicines comprised substances derived from plants, minerals, or other natural sources that had empirically been found to possess therapeutic qualities. In some cases, as with purging agents, the therapeutic effect was based on their mythical ability to expel certain bad humors or toxins from the body. While this attribute may have had some benefit in select poisonings or other intoxications — and still does in some instances today — it clearly had no effect on the course of most infectious diseases. In fact, it may have even caused a worsening in the clinical course of patients with severe infections because it caused them to become further depleted of fluids in their body, hence exacerbating an already depleted state.

The first hundred years of therapy for meningococcal meningitis — before the introduction of serum therapy in the early twentieth century — involved largely symptomatic and "alexipharmic" — antidote — therapies. These included such treatments as "nutritious diet...Peruvian bark and bitters...tincture of iron...twigs of the hemlock tree...brandy, spiced wine, opium and arsenite of potash...calomel, ipecacuanha...cold and tepid ablution...rhubarb"; these specific interventions were recommended for specific symptoms or manifestations of the disease.[1] Although such approaches gave both patients and their physicians at least some

A.W. Artenstein, *In the Blink of an Eye: The Deadly Story of Epidemic Meningitis*,
DOI 10.1007/978-1-4614-4845-7_6, © Springer Science+Business Media New York 2013

measure to attempt to alleviate the suffering associated with meningitis, they did little to alter the dismal natural history of the disease.

With advances in the field of chemistry came advances in medicine. Although it was widely known that many plants contained medicinal properties, delineation of their specific, active substances eluded science until the tools of technology had progressed to a point that such laboratory experiments could be performed.[2] The bark of cinchona plants—a species native to the tropical forests of South America—was known to have therapeutic properties for malaria and other "tropical fevers" for nearly 300 years before its chemical basis—the alkaloid agent quinine—was discerned in the laboratory.

As the field of synthetic, analytical organic chemistry developed through a series of rapid, incremental advances in the middle and late nineteenth century—in parallel with advances in microbiology, immunology, and other scientific disciplines during that period—researchers transitioned from working to isolate medicinally active substances from natural products to the actual production of these substances through chemical synthesis in the laboratory. The first, major breakthrough in this arena came from experiments with a thick, dark, oily liquid—coal tar—used in the dye industry.

In the spring of 1856, an 18-year-old chemistry assistant, William Henry Perkin, working to synthesize quinine in a makeshift laboratory in his East London home, made the serendipitous discovery that aniline—an organic compound derived from coal tar—could be chemically transformed to produce a brilliant purple pigment. Perkin proceeded to commercialize the pigment—"mauveine"—thus not only becoming a very wealthy young man but also becoming the inadvertent founder of the commercial dye industry.[3]

Early on, the English and French dominated the fledgling dye industry. But aided by lax or absent patent laws, Germany rapidly ascended to primacy in the field, a situation formalized with the founding of Friedrich Bayer & Co.—later Bayer—in Barmen, Germany by dye salesman Friedrich Bayer and dyer Johann Weskott in 1863. Soon after, Bayer had competition—Hoechst dyeworks was founded the same year—followed some years later by Baden Aniline and Soda Factory—BASF.[4-6] The dye industry in Germany quickly became a massive one, spurred by the rapid growth in textile manufacturing—its main market—as a consequence of the Industrial Revolution. Within just a few decades, Bayer had become an international powerhouse in the production of industrial dyes.

The relationship between chemically synthesized dyes and medical science, although perhaps not self-evident, became apparent early in the history of the former. Newly invented dyes advanced the technology of microbial and tissue staining—of great importance to the fledgling field of microbiology—as evidenced in the early work of Paul Ehrlich with methylene blue. But synthetic dyes would contribute much more to the field of medicine than as simple laboratory tools. In the 1880s, the same decade in which Koch discovered the bacterial etiologies of tuberculosis and cholera and in which he laid down the principles for growing bacteria in the laboratory, it became apparent to German industrial chemists that compounds involved in the production of dyes had potential therapeutic value.

The common denominator of dyes and medicines was coal tar. A usually discarded by-product of the carbonization of coal, coal tar was therefore a highly abundant raw material—albeit one without obvious utility—of nineteenth century industrialization. It was also the basis of the first synthetic medicinal compounds. Derivative forms are still used today in various topical and shampoo formulations for skin conditions such as dandruff and psoriasis. Some of the aniline compounds derived from coal tar that were used to synthesize dyes—initially indigo but later other colors as well—were also found, in many cases through serendipity, to have medicinal effects.[7]

The first of these synthetic dyes-turned-medicinal agents was acetanilide, a highly toxic compound with antipyretic—fever-lowering—effects. In 1887, the same year that Weichselbaum identified meningococcal bacteria in patients with meningitis in Vienna, Carl Duisberg—the inaugural research director and later management board chairman of Bayer—devised a method to chemically modify acetanilide, rendering it a less toxic but highly potent antipyretic as well as analgesic.[8] The widespread medicinal use of that compound—phenacetin, the parent drug of acetaminophen—Tylenol®—and its economic ramifications impelled the diversification of the rapidly growing German dye industry into the pharmaceutical research business.

Perhaps the most important landmark in the early history of the commercial pharmaceutical industry, occurring in the final days of the nineteenth century, also involved the relief of pain, headaches, and fevers. The medicinal effects of various extracts of plants, including those from willow tree bark and the meadowsweet herb, were probably known since the time of Hippocrates, the ancient Greek father of modern medicine. A synthetic form of salicylic acid, the medically active ingredient in these homeopathic remedies, first isolated during the rise of analytical chemistry in the mid-1800s, was produced by Bayer scientists in 1897 and sold worldwide under the trade name of "Aspirin" by 1899.[9] This agent, by virtue of its profitability and global appeal, revolutionized and galvanized the nascent pharmaceutical research industry.

Because of its supremacy in the industrial manufacture of dyes and synthetic chemistry, Germany became the leader in medicinal chemistry during the early years of the first quarter of the twentieth century. Bayer was at the forefront, with its production of phenacetin followed by aspirin and other agents, including—for a brief period during the first decade of the new century—heroin, marketed as a cough suppressant until its addictive nature became widely manifest.[10] In large part a response to the effect of forced reparations and other measures levied against German economic interests resulting from their defeat in World War I, the German chemical industry underwent a massive restructuring in 1925. Three of its major companies—Bayer, Hoechst, and BASF—joined with three of its smaller ones to form I.G. Farben, which by the 1930s was one of the world's largest companies.[11] With the merger, German pharmaceutical research not only consolidated its standing but also advanced its reach into the well traveled yet poorly understood world of infectious disease therapeutics.

Ehrlich is credited with coining the term "chemotherapy"—the use of chemical agents to treat germ causes of disease—in the early 1900s in describing his vision to unite advances in two great streams of scientific research of the era: infectious diseases and synthetic organic chemistry.[12] Although "chemotherapy" is now more often synonymous with cancer treatment, Ehrlich specifically used it to refer to the treatment of infection.

His own research in tissue staining techniques placed him squarely in the arena of dye chemistry and led him to postulate that dyes may possess anti-infective properties. Ehrlich also reasoned that the mechanism by which dyes worked involved two distinct components: a binding component of the molecule—which allowed it to fix to certain fabrics or tissues—and a 'business' end of the molecule, allowing it to color the material. Further, his concept of chemotherapy hinged upon the notion of "selective affinity"—the relative predilection of a chemical for a germ instead of host tissue.[12] But it was Ehrlich's co-discovery of an organic arsenical compound, not a dye, with activity against syphilis—"Salvarsan"—that provided the first successful test of the idea of chemotherapy.[13] He died in 1915, shortly after World War I had ignited a firestorm throughout Europe, having led just the opening salvo of the chemical war on microbial germs.

Although certainly advancing the field of industrial chemistry, the Great War did little to advance the prospect of bacterial chemotherapy, as the industry's efforts were focused elsewhere—on fuel and munitions. Despite stuttering attempts at chemically based anti-infective therapy during the 1920s, such as the largely futile efforts using mercury-based chemicals—"mercurochrome"—at Johns Hopkins, it was not until the formation of I.G. Farben that the scientific concept of bacterial chemotherapy would be approached in a systematic way. The massive company with its intricate, specialized organizational structure, its culture of innovation, and its strengths in medicinal chemistry research derived from the unification of German industrial dye research and pharmaceutical research was well suited to this effort.[5] Work began there in 1926 and within a decade, the results of their research would forever change the face of pharmaceutical science, medicine, and the world.

Heinrich Hörlein, born in the year that Koch isolated the bacillary cause of tuberculosis, had risen in the ranks of corporate science from a staff chemist in the pharmaceutical division at Bayer to manager of Bayer's pharmaceutical research laboratories before becoming one of I.G. Farben's research managers and director of the pharmaceutical research efforts there after the merger. He was a company man, operating not only with a clear understanding of the process of scientific discovery but also with an even clearer appreciation for the precedence of patents and profits over pure intellectual pursuits.[5] Part of his domain involved the nexus between chemistry and medical research at I.G. Farben, and he focused the efforts in these arenas towards the problem of anti-infective chemotherapy.

The research team for the chemotherapy efforts at I.G. Farben included two dye chemists—Fritz Mietzsch and Joseph Klarer, both working in the area of azo dyes and their potential as antimalarials—and Gerhard Domagk, a research physician who had witnessed firsthand the human cost of infections during his service, as a medical student, on the western front during World War I.[14] After becoming a medical doctor, Domagk embarked on an academic career studying bacterial infections. In 1927, he became the director of a laboratory in experimental pathology within the pharmaceutical research division under Hörlein, although he continued to consider himself an academic—a stance that would affect him for the rest of his career there.

Among Domagk's earliest efforts in industry was the development of an animal model for streptococcal infections, the latter a cause of some of the most dangerous infections of the time, including wound infections and childbed—puerperal—fever. The importance of animal models in understanding disease processes was a long-standing tenet of German pathologic anatomy research dating back to the nineteenth century, emphasized by perhaps the most renowned of all German pathologists— Rudolf Virchow.[15] The reliance at I.G. Farben on rigorous testing of candidate chemical compounds in laboratory animals would run them afoul of the National Socialist—Nazi—movement in Germany, a burgeoning political power whose ideology included an extreme antivivisection credo.

In a process that was far ahead of its times and would presage modern-day 'Big Pharma' procedures, the team at Farben used in vitro—test tube-based—studies to inform their selection of chemical compounds with potential promise that warranted advancement to experimental animal studies. After a series of unsuccessful efforts, the chemists on the team turned their attention back to the azo compounds—key components of industrial dyes with which the company had substantial experience and expertise; they had already exploited this in their pharmaceutical research on novel antimalarial agents, which resulted in the drug Atabrine—a new and improved version of quinine.[5]

By late 1932, Mietzsch and Klarer had prepared hundreds of candidate azo compounds that through in vitro and animal testing had been whittled down to just a few with anti-infective activity in Domagk's lab.[5] In many instances in scientific discovery, there is a 'moment'—a final step or analytic revelation, usually undertaken to solve an experimental problem or advance a thesis, that turns out—although generally only in retrospect—to be defining. Often, the revelation is based on serendipity. Examples of this phenomenon abound. Flexner, as we previously learned, had his 'moment' with the revelation that intrathecal delivery of antimeningococcal serum was an effective treatment for the disease; Pasteur, as we shall soon discover, had one such 'moment' after bacterial cultures had been inadvertently left on his lab bench during his vacation. For the I.G. Farben, anti-infective, chemotherapy research group, the synthetic addition of a sulfonamide chemical group to the azo dye molecule was their 'moment.'

It had long been known within the chemical dye industry that such substances had to have an affinity for textiles and fabrics in order to render them useful as commercial products. Although the molecular basis for this property was not precisely known, it was known that part of the dye molecule was responsible for attaching to the material and the other part was responsible for the color. Ehrlich, as we have seen, used such reasoning to hypothesize that the affinity of dyes to bind to and stain human or animal tissues could be extrapolated to deliver his envisioned chemotherapy to infected cells.[12]

The pharmaceutical researchers at Farben, steeped in dye chemistry, harnessed their experience to this end. They had earlier shown that resistance of dyes to degradation by sunlight or washing could be enhanced by chemical modification—adding sulfonamide groups to the dye molecules. They subsequently applied this knowledge to synthesize a similar compound for Domagk to test.[16] The resulting product, a chemically modified, sulfonamide-containing azo compound—a red dye—was dramatically effective in curing mice infected with lethal doses of streptococci.[5, 16]

Within days of the crucial animal experiments—Christmas Day 1932—the company filed a patent in Germany for their novel chemotherapeutic dye—Prontosil. Although neither the results of their experiments nor the compounds themselves would be available to the general scientific community for more than two years—patents and potential profits trumped publication, as they do in today's pharmaceutical industry—the potential impact of the new invention was immediately clear. For the first time, "a breach had been created in the ramparts of bacterial diseases".[16] This new class of compounds with therapeutic activity against human bacterial infections would revolutionize the treatment of many of the most common causes of illness and death.

As with many momentous discoveries in science, controversy as well as promise surrounded Prontosil. But it was not so much wrangling over who deserved or received credit for the invention—although certainly an element of this did,emerge later—as it was the intrusion of politics into science. Such incursions were not new to the German medicinal chemistry industry. A half a century after the invention of Bayer's "drug of the century"—Aspirin—Arthur Eichengrün, a Jewish chemist working at Bayer at that time, challenged Felix Hoffman's claim of priority for the discovery, claiming that his own role had been censored from company documents by Nazi historical revisionists.[9] But the political circumstances surrounding the invention of Prontosil were unique in the annals of history.

A month after the patent had been filed, Hitler ascended to the position of Chancellor, marking the beginning of the Third Reich and accelerating his reign of terror that darkly colored German history for subsequent decades. Nazi influences, policies, and ideologies suffused and probably hindered anti-infective pharmaceutical research at I.G. Farben. The Nazi regime viewed scientific medicine as elitist and corporate, placing profits ahead of the health of the German people and favoring professional specialists over traditional German folk healers.[5]

As with most elements of Hitler's ideology, anti-Semitism had a position of prominence; Jews were somehow at the root of all that was anti-German. Naturally, this vitriol extended to scientific medicine. Nazi propaganda of the time lampooned and demonized the great advances of the era—many of them by renowned German citizens who were celebrated elsewhere—such as "the Jew Behring" and his serum therapy for infectious diseases and "the Jew Ehrlich" and his Salvarsan therapy for syphilis.[5]

Animal research was an early target of the new regime, in keeping with Nazi antivivisectionist leanings. Although animal research activity was stymied at I.G. Farben for a time under the Nazi regime, it was not halted; political maneuverings by Hörlein, including his ill-fated decision to join the Nazi Party—one that would have detrimental consequences for him at Nuremberg after World War II—and others successfully allowed its continuation.

Other Nazi edicts had far-reaching effects. Domagk spent a week in prison for his unofficial acceptance of the Nobel Prize in Physiology or Medicine in 1939 based on his invention of Prontosil. Hitler had forbidden Germans to accept any such prizes after an opponent of the regime had been awarded the Nobel Peace Prize a few years earlier.[17] Domagk did not officially receive the Nobel until after the War; in a noteworthy slight, his chemistry colleagues, Mietzsch and Klarer, went unrecognized by the Committee.[18] Even in its aftermath the Third Reich continued to impact research at I.G. Farben. Of the two dozen I.G. Farben-employed defendants, among them Heinrich Hörlein, more than half were convicted of war crimes at Nuremburg for their roles in facilitating the war effort through their development of alternative energy sources and poison gas—Zyklon B—as well as for their use of concentration camp slave labor.[19]

Notwithstanding the political maneuvering, appeasement, and lobbying necessitated by a ruling government hostile to scientific medical research, work on Prontosil and its second-generation derivatives continued—with great success at I.G. Farben. And once word of the carefully guarded company secret leaked out—initially with the publication of the French patent in 1934 but more universally with Domagk's first publication of the research findings one year later—scientists in other countries expeditiously embarked on their own laboratory and clinical studies. Prontosil proved highly effective in clinical studies of bacterial infections in humans, including skin and soft tissue infections, throat infections—including a high profile one in U.S. President Franklin Delano Roosevelt's son, childbed fever and other gynecologic infections, and bloodstream infections caused by streptococci. Its successes were widely reported in the scientific literature as well as the lay press of the time.[20–22]

A number of other, novel chemotherapeutic agents based on the "sulfa" moiety were introduced in rapid succession over the subsequent five years. Developed by the French later in 1935, sulfanilamide—the colorless, active constituent of the dye-based Prontosil—possessed enhanced antibacterial activity and less toxicity than its parent drug. Thus, the field turned its attention to this chemical fragment of Prontosil; the child displaced the parent and henceforth, antibacterial drug development pursued a path of chemical modifications of this core to produce other, even more broadly effective sulfa derivatives in Germany, France, England, and the United States.[5, 23]

The widespread production and use of the sulfa-based anti-infective agents had a transformative and immediate effect on the treatment of many, distinct infectious diseases. Other than serum therapy for select diseases—a mode of treatment that was difficult to acquire in many areas, cumbersome to employ, and could be fraught with complications—there was no uniformly effective treatment for infections such as lobar pneumonia, among the most common and most lethal diseases of the early twentieth century prior to the introduction of sulfa drugs into clinical practice in the late 1930s. The impact of the new antibacterial drugs was so profound as to render serum therapy almost obsolete overnight. Over the five years or so after the introduction of these agents, their favorable effects had also been reported in clinical trials of various forms of bacterial meningitis, anthrax, endocarditis—an infection of the heart valves, gas gangrene—a leading cause of combat-associated wound infection and death, dysentery, gonorrhea, and ear and eye infections.

Although its mechanism of antibacterial action remained unknown for a decade, the effect of sulfa drugs on disease-associated death rates was indisputable. Case fatality rates from puerperal fever dropped from twenty-five percent to eight percent, a drop of nearly two-thirds; and those from pneumococcal pneumonia, one of the greatest killers of the time, dropped by a similar magnitude.[23] The effect on gonorrhea—not a lethal disease but one of high morbidity—misery—was equally as impressive. And the impact of these new "miracle drugs" extended to the entire, nascent pharmaceutical industry. A tragic cluster of deaths due to a sulfanilamide "elixir" contaminated with diethylene glycol—a poisonous organic solvent used in the production of resins and explosives—in Oklahoma in 1937 led to passage of the first legislation that mandated formal toxicity testing on new drugs in the United States and permanently changed the focus of government regulation of the industry.[24]

The treatment of meningococcal meningitis was also revolutionized by the advent of the sulfa drugs.[25] Beginning in 1937 with the recognition that sulfanilamide was an effective chemotherapeutic agent for the disease, meningitis mortality rates showed dramatic declines. The death rate—roughly eighty percent in the nineteenth century without specific treatment—had dropped to thirty percent with meningococcal antiserum; with sulfa, it dropped again to less than ten percent.[23] By the onset of World War II, sulfa-based therapy was an established therapeutic regimen for meningococcal meningitis within the U.S. Army. Shortly thereafter, newer generation sulfa agents were routinely being used for chemoprophylaxis as well—to prevent disease by treating asymptomatic carriers of the germ.

The novelty of sulfa drugs was short lived; a mere eight years after their invention had been announced to the world, a team of researchers in Oxford had rediscovered the potential antibacterial powers of the mold *Penicillium notatum*, that had been first recognized—serendipitously—by Alexander Fleming at St. Mary's Hospital in London in 1928.[26] After successfully navigating years of laboratory experiments and thorny production problems with the novel, chemically active substance derived from the fungus, Howard Florey, Ernst Chain, Norman Heatley, and their team at Oxford University had arrived at the stage where the nascent antibacterial drug could be pressed into action—where it was urgently needed—in the North African theater of World War II. There, and elsewhere, penicillin proved highly effective. By the latter years of the War, penicillin had largely replaced sulfa in every infantryman's first-aid kit; by War's end, it had acquired a similar status in the physician's bag.

The invention of sulfa drugs and the discovery of penicillin shortly thereafter unleashed a torrent of antimicrobial drug discovery over the ensuing two decades. For all of their positive attributes for physicians and their patients, the discovery of these drugs also unleashed a certain apathetic outlook within both the lay and medical communities that infectious diseases—entities that had plagued humankind throughout recorded history—"no longer constitute a serious medical problem".[27] The attitude within the medical profession had reached the point at which even the accurate bacteriologic diagnosis of pneumococcal disease—Osler's aptly described, turn-of-the-century, "captain of the men of death"—was being abandoned because of the ready availability of antimicrobial drugs effective against this pathogen. As we shall see later, the false—as it turned out—sense of complacency engendered by new and effective antimicrobial agents also hindered progress in vaccine science during the same, two-decade period in mid-century. But waiting in the wings was another, even darker downside to the liberal use of antimicrobial drugs.

Charles Darwin, the nineteenth century English naturalist, described the driving force behind the concept of adaptive evolution among finches and other birds of the Galapagos Islands; "natural selection" referred to the process by which those individuals better suited to survive in a particular environment were more likely to reproduce and pass these helpful traits on to their offspring.[28] This struggle for survival is a fact of life. It plays out continuously between populations within a species and between different species, especially under resource-poor, challenging conditions. This concept of "survival of the fittest"—in which "fitness" refers to an organism's reproduction potential not its strength or prowess—is not lost on bacteria and other microbes. The germs that cause infections must undergo constant change to ensure their survival in the challenging environments of their human and animal hosts.

A mere decade after the introduction of sulfa drugs, resistance to these agents among gonococci and certain streptococci was already rampant.[29] *Staphylococcus aureus*—the cause of serious "Staph" infections of skin, bones, joints, bloodstream, and other vital organs—was reported to harbor penicillin resistance less than one year after the drug's introduction; within five years, the majority of isolates were resistant.[30] In a survey of antibiotic resistance among bacteria written in 1955—less than twenty years after the invention of the first antibacterial chemotherapeutic agent—Max Finland, Chief of the Harvard Medical Service at Boston City Hospital and one of the founding fathers of the field of infectious diseases in the United States, cited more than 550 scientific papers dealing with the emergence of drug resistance among humans and animals given antimicrobial agents to either treat or to prevent infections.[31] As anyone who reads the newspapers knows, that problem has only continued to grow and with it, the looming possibility of revisiting a time where bacteria routinely won the struggle for survival.

Meningococci, to some extent, resisted the resistance trends of other bacteria in the immediate aftermath of antimicrobial drug introduction; however, by the mid-1960s, sulfa-resistant strains were commonly encountered.[32] Outbreaks of sulfa-resistant, meningococcal meningitis were soon reported in the United States and elsewhere—in both military and civilian populations.[33–36] From the "alexipharmic" and symptomatic attempts at therapy in the nineteenth century through the deployment of "Flexner's serum" in the early portion of the twentieth century, the outlook for meningococcal meningitis had improved, but it still remained a highly lethal disease. The introduction of potent antibacterial drugs in the 1930s and 1940s promised to turn that tide, yet the aftermath of their widespread use left a promise unfulfilled.

By the late 1960s, it was becoming increasingly clear that "chemotherapy" would not be the ultimate solution to epidemic meningitis. For that, a disease prevention approach drawing on thousands of years of empiric observation and nearly 200 years of direct experience would be needed. Such a strategy—vaccination—would harness the body's own defense mechanisms to ward off would-be infectious threats.

Chapter 7
A Brief History of Vaccines

Heading almost due west from London, the train passes city outskirts and urban fringe housing before the landscape becomes progressively more suburban, replete with upscale homes for those commuting between Bristol and the capital. Travel slightly farther north, and the surroundings quickly become quite rural. Here, within Gloucestershire County, approximately 150 kilometers from London, lying in the valley formed by the east bank of the River Severn, is the 1,200-year-old, bucolic town of Berkeley. Being there, one feels immediately transported back to an earlier time—the eighteenth century—in which local medical practitioners like Edward Jenner rode on horseback to their appointed rounds, gathering afterwards for informal discussions of their cases at The Ship tavern—itself already 200 years old at the time—over lunch and beer.

Although he was not the most famous resident of Berkeley when he returned there in 1773—King Edward II was murdered at Berkeley Castle in 1327—Jenner would later become the town's favorite son. As was customary for aspiring physicians in the early eighteenth century, Jenner apprenticed with rural practitioners throughout his teenage years before going to London in 1770 to study for three years under John Hunter, the master surgeon and physiologist, at St. George's Hospital.[1] That Hunter placed high value on experimental science—so much so that he acquired both gonorrhea and syphilis in the course of self-experimentation—was illustrated in his mentorship of Jenner.[2] Based on Hunter's sage advice—"why think, why not trie [sic] the Expt."—Jenner pursued a number of interests in natural science in addition to medicine; he was elected to Fellowship in the Royal Society in 1789—not for medical research—but for his observations involving the nesting behaviors of the hatchling cuckoo.[3]

Smallpox—"variola"—the most historically significant infectious disease in terms of overall human deaths and social impact—was a major source of morbidity and mortality in Jenner's time. Variolation—the deliberate inoculation of pus or scabs from smallpox-infected individuals into healthy ones in order to produce a localized form of infection—appeared to afford some protection against full-blown disease and had been practiced sporadically for more than a century in various parts of the world including Egypt, Africa, India, and China.[4] It was introduced into the West—England—by Lady Mary Wortley Montagu, the wife of the British Ambassador to the Ottoman Court, in 1721.

However, acceptance of variolation was limited in England due its high rate of complications, substantial death rate—albeit significantly lower than that of naturally acquired smallpox, cost, and risk of contagion. Although variolation was used to quell a smallpox epidemic in colonial Boston and later to prevent outbreaks in General Washington's Continental Army, there remained an urgent need for a safe, broadly applicable method of smallpox prevention. Enter Jenner—then living in a rural, farming town with more cows than people.

The dairy cow was of critical economic import in eighteenth century English agricultural communities. The "Old Gloucester" breed, reddish mahogany in color with variable white markings and a white stripe on its back was built for dairy work—yielding an average of 500 gallons of milk per day in Jenner's time.[5] Although the Gloucester had probably grazed in Berkeley for half a millennium, the animal was on the verge of achieving fame for something only peripherally related to its primary use—the lesions, due to the disease cowpox, that affected its udder and teats, would be the future basis of immune protection against smallpox. For this feat, Pasteur suggested that the term "vaccination," derived from *vacca*—Latin for cow, be used to describe immunization against any infection, nearly a century after that animal played a pivotal role in the development of smallpox vaccine.

The potential protective effect of cowpox against smallpox was the stuff of well-known, popular lore among English farmers. Milkmaids generally had unblemished complexions, presumably protected from the scarring caused by smallpox blisters by virtue of a previous bout with cowpox on their hands—acquired from milking infected cows. Benjamin Jesty, a tenant farmer in Yetminster, turned such anecdotes into action in 1774, inoculating his wife and two children with material acquired from cowpox lesions using stocking needles during a local smallpox outbreak; his act—although controversial in the small town—may have protected the trio and eventually led to Jesty being credited as the "pioneer vaccinator against smallpox".[6] Jenner would have known about the folklore surrounding the preventive properties of cowpox, and his "Hunterian" training in the scientific method may have influenced him to experimentally study the concept.[7]

With this background, Jenner prepared a systematic study of the issue. He published his findings—*An Inquiry into the Causes and Effects of the Variolae Vaccinae, a Disease Discovered in Some of the Western Counties of England, Particularly Gloucestershire, and Known by the Name of the Cow Pox*—at his own expense in 1798, after an initial paper had been rejected by the Royal Society.[8] The work contains a series of twenty-three case histories—some involving more than one individual and others based solely on second-hand knowledge—detailing epidemiological as well as experimental evidence of the protective effect of cowpox against smallpox.[9] Natural cowpox infection of seventeen individuals prevented their subsequent successful variolation—in one case more than forty years later; two individuals with previous cowpox infection resisted smallpox upon exposure to active cases of the disease.

The remaining case histories in the *Inquiry* comprised Jenner's uncontrolled inoculation experiments using cowpox. These involved some of the most memorable characters—human and bovine—in vaccine history. Using material obtained from a "large pustulous sore" on the hand of dairymaid Sarah Nelmes, who had been infected by milking "Blossom," an Old Gloucester breed of cow, he inoculated James Phipps, a healthy 8-year-old neighborhood boy via two superficial incisions on the arm in May 1796. Six weeks later—a month after the boy had recovered from the acute cowpox infection—Jenner variolated him in standard fashion and noted a stereotypical lesion on the arm, but no systemic response.

In 1798, after a hiatus necessitated by a lack of infected animals in the community and following a fortuitous outbreak of cowpox among the local dairy farms that provided more material for study, Jenner again carried out a series of similar vaccinations in children. In these 'experiments,' he not only demonstrated resistance to subsequent variolation in some cases but also showed that cowpox—the immunizing agent—could be successfully transmitted from arm to arm through successive generations. This latter finding raised the possibility—still years away from reality—of vaccination without the continuous need for an animal intermediary.

Jenner's *Inquiry* provided the first experimental data to support the popular belief that cowpox infection represented a potentially viable and safer alternative to variolation for the prevention of smallpox. Perhaps most significantly, it represented the first scientific study of the use of an altered form of an infectious agent of animals to provide cross-protection against a related, human pathogen. Jenner's observations were subsequently confirmed and extended by a variety of investigators and by the early part of the nineteenth century, the concept had disseminated throughout Europe and into the United States—with millions vaccinated. Jenner had opened the door to vaccination; 85 years later, Pasteur would step through it.

While Jenner exploited observations from nature to develop a means of vaccine prevention, Pasteur extrapolated observations from the laboratory towards the same end. In an ironic nod to his own axiom concerning chance favoring the prepared mind, Pasteur serendipitously discovered the phenomenon of attenuation—weakening of microorganisms through laboratory manipulation—and envisioned this as a vaccine strategy.

In 1879, he observed that after successive generations of serial passage in culture—in the presence of elevated temperatures and oxygen—the chicken cholera bacillus—now known as *Pasteurella* spp.—lost its capacity to cause death when injected into chickens. Because chickens were a scarce laboratory resource, Pasteur was forced to recycle the same animals in subsequent experiments using freshly passed and highly virulent strains of bacteria. Remarkably, the chickens that had previously been exposed to and survived injection with the weakened—attenuated—bacilli also survived infection with virulent strains; however, naïve chickens—those that had not been previously exposed to the weaker bacilli—rapidly died upon challenge.[10] He surmised that the attenuated bacteria induced protection in the animal, allowing it to survive a challenge from virulent forms of the same bacteria.

Pasteur, always prescient, recognized that such laboratory-induced "artificial attenuation" could replace the difficult task of identifying naturally attenuated microorganisms, such as Jenner's cowpox. He also understood that this phenomenon would revolutionize vaccine science, and this it did, initiating a new epoch in the battle against communicable diseases—one in which the microbiology laboratory performed a pivotal function. Armed with such knowledge, Pasteur rapidly developed effective, attenuated vaccines against anthrax—a zoonotic disease of immense economic importance at the time—in 1881 and rabies—a frightening and otherwise uniformly lethal disease acquired from the bite of an infected—rabid—animal in 1885. A quarter of a century later, Albert Calmette and Camille Guérin, working at the Institute Pasteur in Lille, returned to the cow as a source for another microbe—a bovine strain of tuberculosis—that could be "artificially attenuated" in the laboratory and developed as a vaccine[11] Bacille Calmette–Guérin—BCG—is still in use today in many parts of the world as a relatively effective vaccine against human tuberculosis.

Stimulated by the great leaps forward in vaccine science initiated by Jenner but transformed by his nineteenth century heir—Pasteur—the field rapidly advanced through novel approaches to other important bacterial diseases. Within one year of Pasteur's dramatic success with a live, attenuated rabies vaccine, researchers at the U.S. Department of Agriculture developed a vaccine against the veterinary pathogen hog cholera by inactivating the causative microbe using the application of heat. This technical advance represented the next critical 'moment' in vaccine science. By the waning years of the nineteenth century, effective, heat-killed bacterial vaccines had been developed for a trio of epidemic killers of the era—cholera, typhoid, and plague—to a large extent by disciples of the Pasteur and Koch schools of science.[12]

The next great advance in vaccines, occurring closely on the heels of the development of heat inactivated products, resulted directly from revelations within the newly discovered, rapidly evolving field of immunology. Emil von Behring and Paul Ehrlich, working in Koch's Institute in Berlin in the 1890s, demonstrated that factors present in the serum were able to prevent death from tetanus and diphtheria—lethal bacterial diseases known to result from the destructive activities of potent protein toxins produced by the microbe.

Behring extended the work to show that the serum "antitoxin" he produced by injecting animals with sublethal doses of tetanus or diphtheria bacilli could be transferred to other animals—allowing them to be protected against the otherwise deadly effects of the bacteria without having to be exposed.[13] For proving this concept of "passive transfer" of immunity, Behring received the inaugural Nobel Prize for Medicine or Physiology in 1901; he also established the principles of serum therapy for infectious diseases that Simon Flexner would adopt five years later for the treatment of epidemic meningococcal meningitis, as we saw earlier.

Behring's antitoxin work and Ehrlich's invention of "toxoids"—inactivated forms of the bacterial toxins—would lead, albeit indirectly, to a novel approach to immunization—toxoid vaccines. However, this advance would take more than twenty-five years and would only be made possible by concurrent developments in Europe's basic chemistry laboratories. Nonetheless, by the early 1930s, effective toxoid vaccines were in use to prevent diphtheria and tetanus. It was not long before tetanus toxoid proved its mettle on the battlefields of World War II; its deployment in Allied forces nearly eradicated tetanus as a cause of morbidity and mortality among combat troops.

By the close of the nineteenth century, through the developments of microbiology and immunology as distinct and rapidly evolving fields and the transformative efforts of Pasteur, Koch, and their disciples, vaccine science had shown great advances. Different types of effective vaccines had been created for many of the most important bacterial scourges of the time: anthrax, cholera, typhoid, plague, and tuberculosis; additionally, the underlying concept for vaccines against diphtheria, tetanus, and pertussis had been discovered. Smallpox—through Jenner's studies—and rabies—à la Pasteur—were preventable by vaccines. Both of these maladies—like many of the most common and potentially lethal childhood diseases of the time—were actually caused by viruses, not bacteria, but the existence of the former still remained unknown. Solving this puzzle would represent another defining 'moment' in vaccine history that would stimulate another flurry of landmark discoveries.

At about the same time that Koch published his landmark work on anthrax, 33-year-old Adolf Mayer, a German agricultural chemist, was appointed as the inaugural Director of the Agricultural Experiment Station and Professor of Botany at the new Agricultural School in Wageningen, a small town in the west-central Netherlands near the German border.[14] Beginning in 1879 and for a decade thereafter, Mayer devoted his laboratory effort to an affliction of tobacco plants—one that he had named "tobacco mosaic disease" because of the heterogeneously pigmented spots on the diseased leaves—that had plagued local farmers in the region.

In an attempt to satisfy Koch's postulates of microbial causality for a particular disease, which had already achieved near-dogma status by the time the Director had become seriously engaged in mosaic disease research, Mayer performed the usual array of microbiologic experiments. Although unable to identify bacteria in diseased plants, he replicated the disorder by inoculating healthy plants with sap expressed from the leaves of diseased ones—thus proving transmissibility, a hallmark of bacterial infections. However, unlike bacteria, which were too large to pass through laboratory filters, the agent of mosaic disease remained infectious despite filtration. Mayer not only recognized the novelty of his observations, but he also realized that they could not be reconciled with Koch's postulates. He therefore characterized the etiologic agent in 1882 as a "soluble, possibly enzyme-like contagium".[15]

Mayer shared his findings with a younger colleague at the Agricultural School, Martinus Beijerinck, a chemist with an interest in botany with whom Mayer had founded the local Natural Science Society.[14] Upon reviewing Mayer's experimental data and performing additional experiments, Beijerinck was also unable to demonstrate the presence of microbes—attributing this to his lack of expertise in microbiology. Although Mayer would later rethink his "soluble contagium" hypothesis in favor of a bacterial etiology, he remained aware that his findings failed to satisfy the accepted requirements regarding microbial causality.

Six years after the publication of Mayer's definitive treatise on tobacco mosaic disease and nearly 2,300 kilometers northeast of Wageningen, a young botanical sciences student, Dimitri Ivanowsky, presented his own research on epidemic mosaic disease to the Academy of Sciences of St. Petersburg, Russia. Like Mayer, he demonstrated the "filterable" nature of the transmissible disease and appropriately concluded that the filtrate was infectious.[16] But also like Mayer, he too interpreted his findings within the confines of the scientifically accepted but restrictive context of Koch's postulates. Because of this, Ivanowsky proposed that his findings either represented laboratory error due to defective filters, or that they resulted from the presence of other filterable materials, such as bacterial toxins, in the diseased sap.

By 1895, Beijerinck had returned to academics after leaving the Agricultural School for a ten-year stint in industrial microbiology in Delft, the South Holland birthplace of van Leeuwenhoek, one of the founding fathers of microbiology. During his first years at the Technical University of Delft, Beijerinck resumed the research on tobacco mosaic disease that he had started years earlier in collaboration with Mayer. Even then, he had appreciated that while the affliction was microbial in nature, it was "not caused by microbes yet discovered".[17] Beijerinck's investigations at Delft proved definitive; he not only confirmed the infectivity of the *contagium vivum fluidum*—soluble living germ—despite filtration, but he importantly demonstrated that unlike bacteria, the culprit of tobacco mosaic disease of plants was incapable of independent growth, requiring the presence of living, dividing host cells in order to replicate.[17]

By building upon the works of Mayer and Ivanowsky with his own, expanded investigations, Beijerinck definitively established that a member of a new class of infective agents—one that would come to be known as viruses—caused tobacco mosaic disease. But largely because of extant dogma—Koch's postulates—it took nearly two decades, beginning with Mayer's work, for the scientific world and the investigators themselves to accept this novel truth—a recurrent theme in scientific and medical discovery.[18] However, once established, their discovery unleashed a torrent of scientific investigation that as with Pasteur and Koch a generation earlier, again revolutionized medicine.

By the end of the first quarter of the twentieth century—essentially the same interval that it took to recognize the existence of viruses and their involvement in tobacco mosaic disease of plants—more than 65 diseases of animals and humans, including rabies, had been attributed to these filterable agents.[19] Furthermore, the fledgling field of virology, launched by the work of the three botanical scientists, laid the foundations that ushered in the "golden age of vaccines."

But before there could be a gilded time, there were a host of technical problems associated with these new microbial agents—viruses—that had to be overcome in order to render them amenable to study in the microbiology laboratory. First, they were very small—much more so than bacteria—making them invisible by standard microscopy. And perhaps most importantly, viruses were obligate parasites; they required living host cells in order to replicate, and thus could not be grown on the standard nutrient media in use in early twentieth century microbiology laboratories.

The ability to cultivate—grow—microbial organisms in the laboratory was, and to some extent still is an essential part of the laboratory study of infectious diseases. It is an important component of diagnosis, clinical understanding, and the development of preventive approaches—such as vaccines. Although in some circumstances, current molecular approaches can replace the need to grow an organism in culture, the latter still remains the gold standard for investigation. Certainly this was the case in the earlier part of the twentieth century. Koch devoted a large portion of his career to solving the technical dilemmas of early bacteriology; much of the second quarter of the twentieth century was spent in similar pursuits within the burgeoning field of virology.

Ernest Goodpasture, a Johns Hopkins trained pathologist who would later return to his native Tennessee and spend the majority of his illustrious career at Vanderbilt, was responsible for one of the earliest and most important technical advancements in experimental virology. In 1931, he demonstrated that certain viruses could be grown on the chorioallantoic membranes of chick embryos—a medium that was originally the domain of embryologists but exploited by cancer researchers at the Rockefeller Institute beginning in 1911.[20] Chorioallantoic membranes are vascular coverings of the egg that are akin to the placenta of mammals. Goodpasture's technical revelations galvanized research with a number of different viruses, including the causes of influenza and yellow fever—leading directly to effective vaccines against both of these pathogens.[21]

The great step forward of growing viruses in embryonic chickens was soon leap-frogged by another great technical advance—tissue culture—spurred on by the efforts of John Enders, a late-bloomer to microbiology who would leave an indelible imprint on the field of virology. At the newly established Research Division of Infectious Diseases at Boston Children's Hospital in the late 1940s, Enders and his young protégés—Tom Weller and Frederick Robbins, physician scientists working in his laboratory—expanded on the idea of growing viruses in living cultures of animal tissue cells, a concept pioneered 40 years earlier in the realms of zoology and tissue preservation.[21] Techniques of tissue culture had been subsequently improved through incremental modifications before being applied to the study of viruses during the two decades preceding Enders' involvement.

The Enders lab harnessed all of the most advanced technologies of the time in their pursuit to propagate viruses for prolonged periods of time in tissue culture. They showed some measure of early success with both mumps—the cause of the common childhood disease—and vaccinia virus—the active component of small-pox vaccines. Then came the big breakthrough. Following the classic Pasteurian axiom that scientific fortune tends to favor disciplined, meticulous, and focused investigators, Weller—as an add-on to another, unrelated experiment—inoculated cultures of aborted human embryonic tissue with a virulent strain of poliovirus that happened to be in Enders' laboratory freezer. Subsequent sampling of the tissue yielded live poliovirus; he had—for the first time—grown poliovirus in tissue culture. The cultivation of polio in this way was not only novel but also proved to be a monumental discovery that resulted in nearly immediate dividends.[22]

For decades, polio had been erupting in periodic and devastating epidemics in the United States and elsewhere. It was not only an important cause of morbidity and mortality among children and young adults, but it also terrorized communities, leaving permanent scars—in the form of paralysis or the need to use a machine to breath—an "iron lung"—long after the acute infection abated.[23] The ability to grow the virus in nonneural tissue culture led directly to the successful attenuation of the virus through serial tissue culture passages. And this—as Pasteur showed with chicken cholera and rabies 70 years earlier—was the penultimate, significant step leading to the development of vaccines.

Just five years after their landmark publication on growing poliovirus in tissue culture the trio—Enders, Weller, and Robbins—was awarded the Nobel Prize for their work. One year later, in 1955, an inactivated poliovirus vaccine developed by Jonas Salk was shown to protect children against the disease and was almost immediately licensed for widespread use.[23] The "golden age of vaccines" had begun. Within fifteen years, effective vaccines against measles, mumps, and rubella—other scourges of childhood—had been developed.

By the late 1960s, "vaccinology"—the term coined by Salk to describe the multifaceted science of vaccines—had become a highly productive pursuit. In the 175 years between Jenner's homegrown experiments with cowpox and the routine use of vaccines against some of the most common childhood pathogens, many infectious diseases—bacterial and viral—had been prevented or brought under control through the use of live, attenuated vaccines, inactivated vaccines, or those derived from detoxified bacterial proteins. However, some of the most important bacterial killers of the time still eluded a vaccine solution, and attention to these pathogens would launch a new era of vaccines.

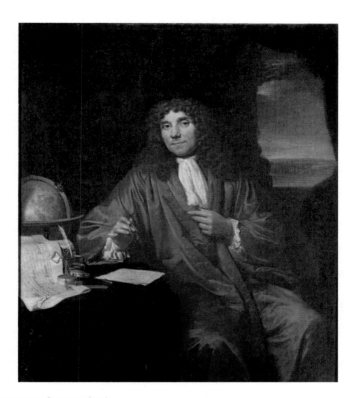

Fig. 1 Antony van Leeuwenhoek

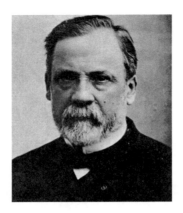

Fig. 2 Louis Pasteur

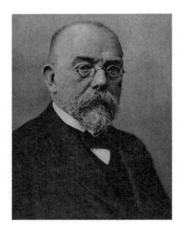

Fig. 3 Robert Koch

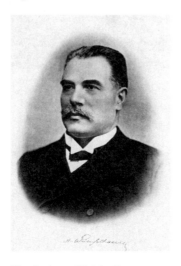

Fig. 4 Anton Weichselbaum

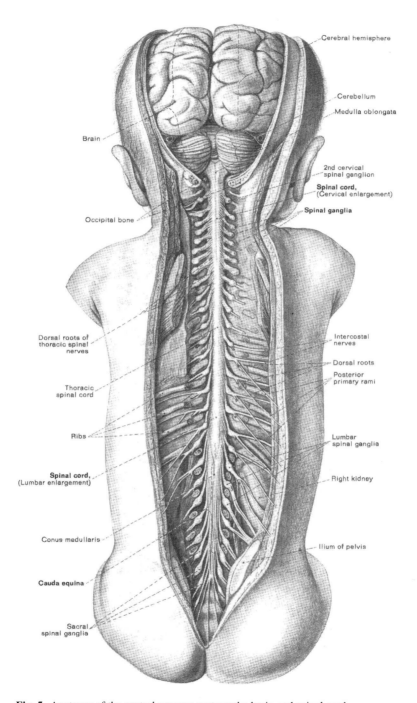

Fig. 5 Anatomy of the central nervous system: the brain and spinal cord

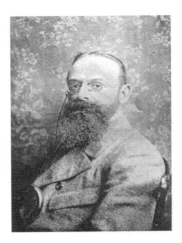

Fig. 6 Albert Neisser

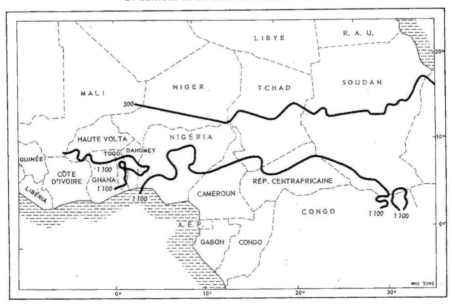

Fig. 7 Lapeyssonnie's original map of the African "meningitis belt"

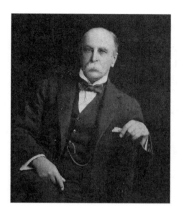

Fig. 8 Sir William Osler

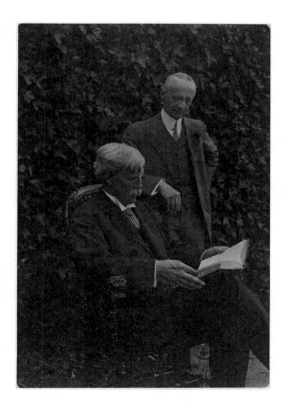

Fig. 9 Simon Flexner (standing) and Frederick Gates

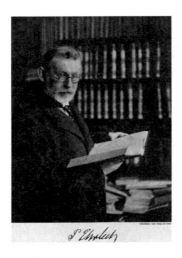

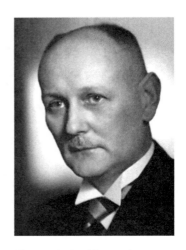

Fig. 10 Paul Ehrlich

Fig. 11 Gerhard Domagk

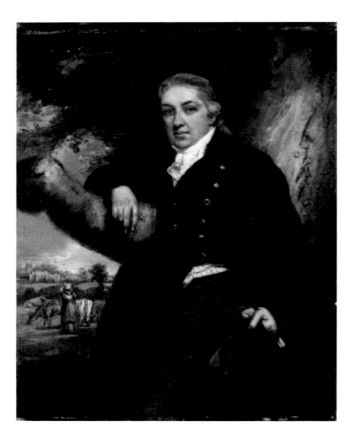

Fig. 12 Edward Jenner

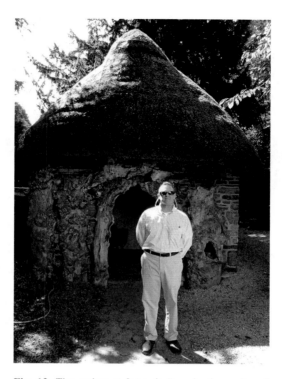

Fig. 13 The author at Jenner's "vaccination cottage," Berkeley, England

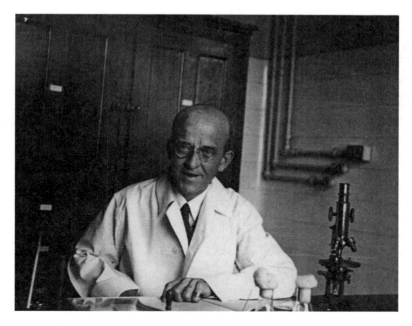

Fig. 14 Oswald Avery

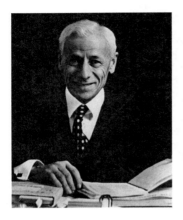

Fig. 15 Michael Heidelberger

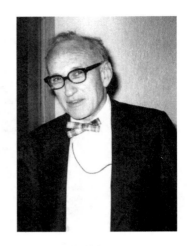

Fig. 16 Elvin Kabat

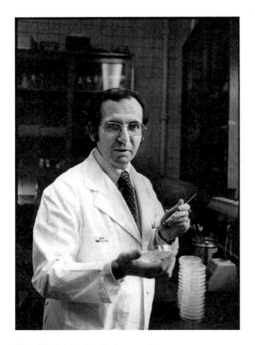

Fig. 17 Malcolm S. Artenstein

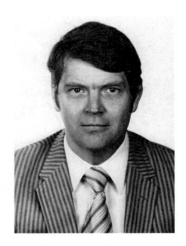

Fig. 18 Emil Gotschlich

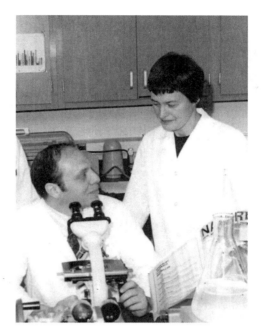

Fig. 19 Irving Goldschneider (seated) and Martha Lepow

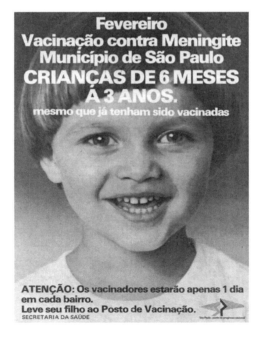

Fig. 20 Poster advocating meningococcal vaccination for children between the ages of 6 months and 3 years in Saõ Paulo, Brazil, 1972

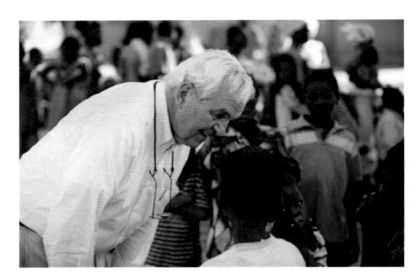

Fig. 21 F. Marc LaForce

Chapter 8
That Soluble Specific Substance

Bacterial infections, as we have seen, remained a cause of significant morbidity and mortality well into the first half of the twentieth century. They remain so today, although the worst culprits are now those acquired not in daily life but in hospitals and other health care facilities. But it is important to remember that neither prevention nor control of bacterial diseases became a possibility until the end of the nineteenth century. Prior to that time, infected individuals either survived—largely on the basis of their intrinsic host defense systems and good fortune—or they succumbed—an outcome that was frighteningly common, even with seemingly trivial infections.

Some bacterial infections, such as anthrax in livestock and the toxin-mediated human diseases diphtheria and tetanus, became largely preventable by the latter part of the nineteenth and early part of the twentieth centuries, respectively, with the use of effective vaccines. Others, such as typhoid and cholera, were largely banished from the developed world by a combination of improvements in hygiene and sanitation, in spite of partially effective vaccines. Still others, such as streptococcal infections, which were highly lethal prior to the late 1930s, were largely controlled by the introduction of sulfa drugs and then penicillin. These and the other newly developed antimicrobial drugs of the 1940s and 1950s appeared—temporarily as it turned out—to hold the promise that bacterial diseases would no longer threaten human health; a promise that, as we have seen, quickly went unfulfilled with the widespread development of drug resistance.

Perhaps the most common and fearsome acute bacterial disease of the early twentieth century was lobar pneumonia—a serious infection of the lungs—caused by a form of streptococcus known as the "pneumococcus." Osler, author of the definitive textbook of medicine of the era—the book that convinced Rockefeller's right-hand man for philanthropy, Frederick Gates, of the necessity for establishing a medical research institute in the United States—devoted nearly 400 pages of his 1000-page, first edition text—forty percent—to descriptions of known or suspected infectious diseases; a significant portion of these involved one entity—pneumonia.[1]

A.W. Artenstein, *In the Blink of an Eye: The Deadly Story of Epidemic Meningitis*,
DOI 10.1007/978-1-4614-4845-7_8, © Springer Science+Business Media New York 2013

The infection was neither an epidemic threat nor usually as rapidly and dramatically lethal as meningococcal meningitis. Pneumococcal disease was so highly prevalent—it accounted for nearly 77,000 deaths in the U.S. in 1890, more than half a million when adjusted for today's population—that Osler borrowed a description used by author John Bunyan in the seventeenth century, dubbing it "captain of the men of death"—replacing tuberculosis for that distinction. Entire hospital wards were filled with these cases.

The pneumococcus was initially and independently discovered in 1881 by both Pasteur—in the course of challenging animals with saliva from victims of rabies— and George Sternberg—a military medical officer who would later become the Surgeon General of the U.S. Army, while examining his own saliva. In addition to his elegant bacteriologic studies, Sternberg left two other great legacies: he was responsible for appointing the Yellow Fever Commission, headed by Major Walter Reed, that would go on to determine the route of transmission and the cause of this dreaded disease; and he founded the Army Medical School—later to be known as Walter Reed General Hospital—a pivotal institution in the subsequent chapter of our story.[2] Five years after its discovery Fraenkel, in Germany, identified the pneumococcus as the major cause of acute lobar pneumonia. The name for the microbe was proposed, shortly thereafter, by Weichselbaum—the Austrian Professor of Pathological Bacteriology who one year later would be the first to identify the meningococcus in autopsy specimens from patients who had died from meningitis.

Almroth Wright, the British Army bacteriologist who had been the first to use killed typhoid vaccine on a large scale in troops deployed to India towards the end of the nineteenth century, tried a similar vaccine approach to prevent pneumococcal disease. In 1911, he vaccinated 50,000 South African gold miners—a group of otherwise healthy, young, African men who were known to be at high risk of pneumococcal disease in the overcrowded, hot, humid, germ 'cauldron' that they lived in for months at a time two miles below the earth's surface—with a vaccine derived from heat-inactivated pneumococci.[3] The results were disappointing; this approach to pneumococcal vaccines was subsequently abandoned.

Although microbiologically unrelated, the pneumococcus and the meningococcus share a common feature other than their prominent roles in causing sickness and death—they both reside within a polysaccharide capsule—a structure composed of a series of complex sugar molecules chemically bound together to form a layer that coats the microbe. This coating—capsule—acts as a shield that protects the bacteria from being engulfed and then degraded by specialized cells—"phagocytes"—of the immune system. Serum antibodies that usually neutralize bacteria and thus protect hosts against infection are unable to neutralize encapsulated microbes; to do so requires specific antibodies directed against the capsule. It was this concept of anti-capsular antibodies that would—after a series of landmark scientific developments— initially inform the search for new forms of pneumococcal vaccines and subsequently, for meningococcal vaccines.

Although it was known since Pasteur's time that certain bacteria produced polysaccharides, the notion that these carbohydrate compounds might be effective to induce immune responses was unlikely to have even been considered by Alphonse

Dochez and Oswald Avery at the time they published their paper in 1917 describing the "specific soluble substance" elaborated by pneumococci grown in broth cultures and found in the blood and urine of patients with lobar pneumonia.[4] Avery, a physician scientist trained in bacteriology, had joined the research staff of the Rockefeller Institute Hospital in 1913. The two scientists shared both a nearby apartment and membership on the "Pneumonia Service" — a laboratory devoted to studying the patients with pneumonia at Rockefeller — in the early years of the hospital.[5] Dochez would move on to other research pursuits within infectious diseases — determining the viral etiology of the common cold and the streptococcal etiology of scarlet fever. However, Avery would spend the remaining 30 years of his active research career at Rockefeller studying the pneumococcus — specifically devoted to understanding the organism's biochemistry and its relationship to the pathogenesis of the microbe. This research thread later led to the discovery by Avery and two colleagues — Colin MacLeod and Maclyn McCarty — that DNA, not proteins, encoded genetic information — a career capstone that would revolutionize biology.[6]

The "specific soluble substance" discovered by Avery and Dochez turned out to also be a seminal finding that would chart the course for future studies and lead eventually to an effective vaccine against not only pneumococcal disease but also for meningococcus. A key feature of the soluble material was that it was "type-specific" — referring to the fact that it was recognized only by homologous antipneumococcal serum — serum that contained antibodies directed against the same strain of the bacteria.

Distinct types or "strains" of the same bacterial species can be differentiated from one another by the immunologic reactions that ensue when they are mixed with the liquid, noncellular portion of clotted blood — the serum — from humans or animals infected with the organism. When a specific bacterial type is mixed in a test tube with serum derived from a person who is infected with the same type, the formation of clumps — a process called "agglutination" — proves that the specific germ has been recognized by corresponding antibodies in the patient's serum. Friedrich Neufield, another of Koch's famous assistants, employed such an "agglutination reaction" in 1902, mixing sera from patients with a variety of different pneumococcal cultures; he observed specific agglutination patterns that suggested the existence of at least three distinct types of pneumococci.[7]

As with pneumococci, not all meningococci are alike; at least four, distinct serotypes of these organisms were recognized in the early years of the twentieth century.[8] These were initially classified in variable ways, depending on where the science was performed: English-speaking countries adopted a I, II, III, and IV classification of types; Europeans used an alphabetical — A through D — classification. The number of serotypes, as we shall see, would subsequently expand; their names would become standardized; and their importance in the epidemiology and control of meningococcal infection would become manifest.

Meanwhile, by the 1920s, Avery had embarked on a course of investigation to determine the chemical basis of immunological specificity of the soluble substance that he had derived from pneumococci. The accepted scientific dogma of the era was that proteins conferred immunologic specificity — they, alone, represented the portion of a chemical compound or microbe that attracted the attention of an individual's immune defense system. However, even though the type-specific soluble substance of the pneumococcus appeared to be the target of the immune system's advances, it did not behave like a protein. Heat and certain cellular enzymes inactivated proteins, but the specific soluble substance resisted these threats, raising the hypothesis that this substance represented an example of an entirely novel scientific paradigm. Because that possibility so challenged the existing supremacy of proteins in accounting for immunologic specificity, Avery himself was reluctant to embrace it. He initially invoked alternative theories that either the material comprised some new kind of protein or perhaps was contaminated by proteins.[9]

To decipher the identity of the specific soluble substance yet lacking the chemistry expertise to do so, Avery established a collaboration with Michael Heidelberger, a young organic chemist working in the department of kidney diseases in the same building at Rockefeller.[9] Within a year, they had ascertained that the soluble substances of distinct pneumococcal serotypes actually comprised complex polysaccharides, and that it was these substances which conferred antigenic—immunologic—specificity to the bacteria.[10, 11] This revelation would have a dramatic effect on the field and would create the foundation for novel vaccines against first the pneumococcus and shortly thereafter, the meningococcus.

But as with other unexpected and revolutionary ideas in science, this one too met with considerable, initial skepticism.[9] The nature of scientific progress has been rightly characterized as comprising intervals of "normal science"—incremental advances based on past achievements—punctuated by periods of "game-changing" discoveries that challenge existing dogma and stir up controversy within the scientific community.[12] Once the upheaval subsides, these events lead to paradigm shifts—new directions in thinking—that galvanize further discoveries and in doing so, move science forward. A similar process occurred, as we previously saw, with the discovery of viruses a generation earlier by three botanists in Europe.[13] However, for Avery and Heidelberger, the controversy soon ebbed as large volumes of experimental, confirmatory data emerged from multiple laboratories.

Other approaches to treating the high burden of pneumococcal disease in communities and hospitals had been attempted in the years before Avery's specific soluble substance shifted scientific thinking about the bacteria towards possible new strategies for host protection. The demonstration of multiple pneumococcal serotypes and the qualified successes of Jochmann, Flexner, and others with antimeningococcal serum therapy in the first decade of the twentieth century had led first to the introduction of this approach in pneumococcal pneumonia.

In 1910, Neufeld, at the Koch Institute in Berlin, protected mice using type-specific antisera; 3 years later, Rufus Cole and Dochez from the Rockefeller Institute Hospital reported success using type I pneumococcal antisera to treat patients with pneumonia.[14] Enthusiasm for using serum therapy in pneumococcal disease briefly escalated with the immunochemical revelations of Avery and Heidelberger a decade later. Although it proved useful in some studies, serum therapy never fulfilled its theoretical potential or the initial promise seen in animal studies. As occurred with serum therapy for meningococcal meningitis, this approach was permanently discarded with the advent of clinically effective antibacterial chemotherapy in the late 1930s.

Efforts to harness the immunologic specificity of pneumococcal capsular poly-saccharides to induce protection against disease followed on the heels of Avery and Heidelberger's revelations. Oscar Schiemann and Wolfgang Casper in Berlin dem-onstrated that purified pneumococcal capsular polysaccharides were immuno-genic — caused immune responses — and engendered type-specific protection in mice.[15] Max Finland and colleagues at Boston City Hospital's Thorndike Laboratory extended these findings in the 1930s, paving the way for human trials of polysac-charide-derived vaccines.[16, 17] An outbreak of pneumococcal pneumonia among recruits awaiting deployment at the Army Air Force Technical School in Sioux Falls, South Dakota in the early 1940s provided the setting for what would be the first, definitive clinical trial of this concept. When it was over, the vaccine — contain-ing polysaccharides from the four major pneumococcal serotypes — had proven to be highly successful in preventing type-specific pneumococcal pneumonia among 8,586 troops.[18]

Enthusiasm for the initial success of pneumococcal polysaccharide vaccines would be ephemeral — erased by the new wonders — antimicrobial drugs — that had also replaced serum therapy for both meningococcal meningitis and pneumococcal disease. The introduction of sulfa drugs into clinical practice in the late 1930s and of penicillin a decade later, dramatically improved the prognosis of many of the most common and deadly bacterial diseases of the time. But the availability of these "miracle drugs" also had an unintended effect; it led, as we have seen, to a sense of complacency within the medical and scientific communities regarding infectious threats. Physicians — and society — felt that microbes would be vanquished with these new, powerful weapons. This prevailing attitude would limit polysaccharide vaccine research for years to come.

Despite the availability of the first antibacterial chemotherapy — sulfa drugs, epi-demic meningococcal meningitis remained an important concern as the United States mobilized for war in the early 1940s. The disease was known to cause recur-rent epidemics in Africa in the early part of the twentieth century, and epidemic meningococcal meningitis had erupted in U.S. recruit training camps during World War I, causing nearly 6,000 cases with more than one-third of those resulting in death, despite the use of serum therapy.[19] For these reasons, military leaders included meningococcal disease on the list of "mission relevant" health problems that required attention and planning prior to our involvement in Europe's war.

Such concerns prompted the inception of the Commission on Meningitis as part of the original charter of the Armed Forces Epidemiological Board in early 1941.[20] The Board represented an innovative effort by the Secretary of War to engage the best and brightest experts in civilian, academic medicine and to team them up with their military counterparts in preventive medicine and public health in order to scientifically address some of the most important health risks for the troops as American involvement in World War II seemed increasingly certain. Its original mission specifically revolved around the potential for a catastrophic outbreak of influenza — as had occurred during World War I — but quickly burgeoned into smaller

"Commissions" for the study of other threats: measles, pneumonia, streptococcal infections, other acute respiratory diseases, and viruses of the nervous system. The Commission on Meningitis was among the earliest formed—in February of 1941, nearly a year before the U.S. entered World War II.

Outbreaks of meningococcal disease erupted again during military preparations to enter World War II. By war's end, the U.S. Army had experienced nearly 14,000 cases of meningococcal disease, three-quarters of them occurring among non-deployed troops in the continental U.S.[19] The death rate—four percent—was significantly lower than that seen during the previous war, in large part due to the routine, mandated use of sulfadiazine as prophylaxis for new recruits during the cooler months when acute respiratory diseases were prevalent. However, the total number of deaths—559—and the death rate—the number who died for every 100,000 soldiers, a standardized way to look at deaths between different diseases—was higher for meningococcal disease than for any other infectious disease except for tuberculosis during World War II.

Based on the rapidity with which the disease affected vulnerable individuals during outbreaks and the experience with it during World War I, a preventive approach appeared to be the best strategy for meningococcal disease. Despite this, the concept of preventing outbreaks of meningococcal meningitis using a vaccine approach had not been studied prior to American involvement in World War II. But now, based on the recognition that the specific soluble substance—capsular polysaccharide—of the pneumococcus conferred its immunologic specificity and informed by a number of animal and human studies with pneumococcal polysaccharides in the 1930s, the idea of applying those lessons towards a vaccine for meningococci began to take shape—at least in one laboratory. This would prove to be the only foray into this territory before the widespread use of newly minted antibacterial drugs changed research priorities for more than two decades.

In 1937, the same year that sulfa was shown to be the first effective antimicrobial treatment for meningococcal meningitis, twenty-three-year-old Elvin Kabat was awarded his PhD based on work involving the immunochemistry of antibodies in Heidelberger's laboratory at Columbia, where the great chemist had landed nine years previously after leaving the Rockefeller Institute Hospital.[21] Described by his mentor as a "young whirlwind," Kabat had initially joined Heidelberger's laboratory as a "helper" assigned to routine laboratory chores—including washing the glassware—but his scientific curiosity and prowess were quickly appreciated, as he successfully developed novel methods for the quantitative assessment of bacterial agglutination.[22]

Shortly thereafter, as part of his antibody chemistry work, Kabat demonstrated the presence of meningococcal anticapsular antibodies in the convalescent sera of experimental animals. This finding, along with the ongoing, albeit more advanced efforts with field trials of pneumococcal polysaccharide vaccines at the time—an area in which Heidelberger, his laboratory director, was actively involved—and the start of American military involvement in the war, emboldened him to suggest a preliminary human trial of a homegrown, purified, group A meningococcal polysaccharide vaccine.[22]

The small study, funded by the Commission on Meningitis, was designed to assess whether the vaccine would induce an immune response in 38 medical student volunteers. After only four of the volunteers showed an antibody response to the vaccine, the line of research was not pursued.[23] Kabat would go on to become a leading force in experimental immunology and over the next forty years would train dozens of future leaders in the field—none of whom would revisit meningococcal vaccines.

Further development of meningococcal polysaccharide vaccines at the time suffered the same fate as that of pneumococcal vaccines—relegated to file cabinets by the initial promise of antimicrobial chemotherapy. However, within twenty-five years of their introduction into clinical practice, it was evident that these drugs had failed to halt the inexorable mortality among many patients with severe pneumococcal pneumonia.[24] Additionally, by the early 1960s, it was also clear that another pathogen coated by a polysaccharide capsule—the meningococcus—was still causing significant epidemics. These outbreaks, occurring both in the U.S. and overseas, were increasingly being caused by meningococci that were resistant to the effects of antimicrobial drugs, confirming the clinical importance of drug resistance.[25]

The occurrence of drug-resistant meningococcal disease at military bases and the fully realized specter of another war—Vietnam—for America provided the sparks that would be needed to revitalize interest in preventive approaches to epidemic meningococcal meningitis.[26] The research effort galvanized by these events would build upon the previous work of Avery, Heidelberger, and Kabat and carry it to its logical conclusion—the first effective meningococcal vaccine.

Chapter 9
Towards a Vaccine

As Americans were becoming progressively more deeply involved in Vietnam, first as "advisors" but subsequently in the mid-1960s as full-fledged combatants, the Army Medical Department was developing plans and organizing health priorities in order to fulfill its mission to "conserve the fighting strength." As we have seen, outbreaks of meningococcal meningitis had occurred during both world wars, and the disease remained a significant cause of mortality and lost duty time among recruits at basic training sites in the U.S. in between wars. Additionally, meningitis was known to occur worldwide in both its epidemic and sporadic forms, making it an ongoing health threat wherever the military might deploy in the future.

Because of these concerns, the Army Medical Department made the strategic decision to direct a focused component of its broad research activities in communicable diseases and preventive medicine towards solving the problem of meningococcal meningitis. The staging ground for this work would be at 'command central' for such research in the Army—the Walter Reed Army Institute of Research in Washington, D.C.

Walter Reed General Hospital—built on the site from which Confederate General Jubal Early had attacked the nation's capital in July 1864—opened its doors to ten patients in May 1909. As the namesake of the recently deceased Army officer who had presided over the landmark studies on yellow fever transmission in Cuba, it boasted an 80-bed capacity and the distinction of being the first, named, permanent, Army general hospital.[1]

Sixteen years earlier, in 1893—the same year that Simon Flexner received his first faculty appointment in pathology at Johns Hopkins—Army Surgeon General George Sternberg had established the new Army Medical School on the grounds of the Army Medical Library and Museum in the Southwest quadrant of Washington, D.C.[2] Sternberg, widely considered to be the founding father of American bacteriology, had independently isolated—along with Pasteur—the pneumococcus in 1881, thus endowing him with indirect ties to polysaccharides and the meningococcal vaccine research that would occur nearly a century later within the organization he created.

A.W. Artenstein, *In the Blink of an Eye: The Deadly Story of Epidemic Meningitis*,   75
DOI 10.1007/978-1-4614-4845-7_9, © Springer Science+Business Media New York 2013

The Medical School would move to the northern edge of Washington—to the tree-lined, Takoma Park campus of Walter Reed General Hospital—in 1923. Twenty-eight years later, the hospital and medical school would be officially combined to form the Walter Reed Army Medical Center. In 1953, the medical school ceased to exist as a functioning unit; its research components, housed in the large, H-shaped building 40 on the grounds of the Medical Center, became the Walter Reed Army Institute of Research—WRAIR.

WRAIR and its Army Medical School predecessor already enjoyed a storied scientific history at the time that research on meningococcal vaccines began in earnest there in the latter part of the 1960s. Within its stated mission involving public health and prevention of disease and its inherent global perspective, the list of important medical achievements that derived from that single institution during its first seventy years of existence was unparalleled.

In the early years, before moving to the grounds of the hospital, WRAIR researchers were responsible for significant advances in preventive medicine. The investigations of the Typhoid Board in 1898 and those of the Yellow Fever Commission in Cuba two years later, both commissioned by Surgeon General Sternberg and headed by an Army physician—Major Walter Reed—established critical epidemiologic features of these two diseases, allowing for their eventual control among troops by vaccination. Following these efforts, Major Frederick Russell introduced mass typhoid vaccination of soldiers in 1909. Major Carl Darnell pioneered the use of chlorine to purify drinking water in 1910—forming the basis for future water purification technologies. Lieutenants Charles Craig and Percy Ashburn had proven the viral etiology of dengue fever—a severe tropical infection—in 1907; twenty years later, Colonel Joseph Siler demonstrated that the disease was mosquito borne. And Colonel Edward Vedder showed that the nutritional deficiency affecting peripheral nerves and the heart—beriberi—caused by a lack of vitamin B_1 in the body, can be prevented or treated by ingesting rice bran extract. When the new WRAIR building was completed on the grounds of Walter Reed in 1932, its four named pavilion wings—Sternberg, Vedder, Craig, and Siler—paid homage to some of these early accomplishments.

Because of the importance of communicable diseases to the health of U.S. military members and their dependents, much of the focus of WRAIR's research was trained on these issues. Microbiologist Maurice Hilleman, who would later go on to Merck where he would work for more than 45 years and be responsible for developing and licensing more human vaccines than any other scientist in history, isolated the virus—later named adenovirus—that caused the majority of seasonal, acute respiratory disease outbreaks in military recruit centers.[3] Both Hilleman, and later Ed Buescher—Director of the Division of Viral Diseases—spearheaded successful adenovirus vaccine research at WRAIR. In 1961, Buescher's research team, comprising two young Army physicians, Malcolm Artenstein and Paul Parkman, was one of two groups in the U.S. to simultaneously and independently isolate the rubella virus—the cause of German measles—from patient samples. Their work would lead to the development of an effective, licensed rubella vaccine within a decade. The next great challenge for WRAIR researchers would be to find a way to prevent epidemic meningitis among troops.

The specter of recurrent, epidemic meningococcal disease at military basic training sites—beginning to bustle by the early 1960s with renewed activity in preparation for escalating efforts in Vietnam—was a compelling concern of military planners. Beginning during World War II, short—three-day—courses of the antibacterial drug sulfadiazine were used to prevent meningitis in military recruit camps. The drug worked by eradicating the meningococci from their temporary homes in the noses and throats of soldiers; without carriers, the germ was not passed from one recruit to another—thus, profoundly limiting the opportunity for epidemic disease to ignite. However, as we have seen, within two decades—by the early 1960s—meningococci had become progressively more resistant to the effects of sulfa drugs. This, combined with the increasingly common reports of outbreaks of antibiotic resistant meningococcal meningitis within the U.S. and abroad, intensified the apprehension of military commanders.

A series of highly publicized outbreaks in the U.S. through the early 1960s heightened their discomfort. Distinct but nearly concurrent epidemics of sulfa-resistant group B meningitis occurred at both Army and Navy recruit facilities in California in 1963.[4] The next year, an outbreak at Fort Ord—a massive Army training camp south of San Francisco that housed nearly 30,000 recruits at a time—resulted in 104 cases of meningococcal disease.[5] Most of these occurred in combat trainees, but ten of them affected civilian military dependents; fourteen of these patients died, two of the civilians among them. The Fort Ord outbreak led to such negative press and near "hysteria" in the surrounding communities that the Army was forced to temporarily suspend basic training there—an almost unheard of event in the military.

The impact of these episodes—magnified by further outbreaks among both military and civilian groups in the U.S. and abroad—convinced the U.S. military command that a focused effort against the meningococcus by the Army Medical Department was necessary. Prevention—WRAIR's specialty—was the last best hope, and this meant the development of a meningococcal vaccine. To attain this goal would require a well-reasoned, informed, logical, and organized experimental approach that would draw upon a half century of immunochemistry and polysaccharide research. Buescher knew just who to turn to for this critical project.

Malcolm Artenstein, like most eligible members of the class of 1955 at Tufts University Medical School in Boston, was drafted into the Army. After residency training in internal medicine and a research fellowship in the fledgling discipline of infectious diseases with Louis Weinstein—the prototypical physician–scientist and master teacher in the field—he was called to active duty in 1959. At Fort Sam Houston in Texas, the place where every physician underwent basic training in those days, he was singled out—rarely a positive in the Army—for his infectious diseases credentials and thus brought to the attention of Buescher at WRAIR, who was looking for young talent. Buescher had already been made aware of Artenstein through a conversation with Lou Weinstein. This was a fortuitous occurrence for the young conscript, likely saving him an assignment to some desolate Army clinic or remote field hospital.

Upon arrival at WRAIR, Artenstein immediately became involved in the work on the rubella virus there, culminating in the first report of its isolation.[6] His two-year military obligation ended and never feeling entirely comfortable in uniform—he would cross the street to avoid having to return the salute of enlisted soldiers—Artenstein returned to civilian, academic medicine with Dr. Weinstein in Boston. But this was to be short lived; in 1962, at the age of 32, he was back at WRAIR—as a civilian—after accepting an offer from Buescher that was too good to pass up to be first the Assistant Chief of the Department of Viral Diseases and then, in 1966, the Chief of the Department of Bacterial Diseases. He would remain there for the rest of his brief, but highly productive career.

In those early years back at WRAIR, Artenstein's research focused on viral infections of the respiratory and nervous systems and on mechanisms of immunity against viruses. In 1966, he started working on meningococcal disease. In short order, this work became his singular focus and kept him in the laboratory at least six days during most weeks and reviewing data at home at night. Artenstein was a thoughtful, methodical, yet creative researcher who understood the importance of building and nurturing a strong research team in order to answer the important scientific questions. He had a keen ability to "ask the crucial questions, obtain the critical data, and analyze it objectively"—quickly grasping the potential implications of experimental findings and then designing and executing the appropriate investigations to advance the studies.[7]

Artenstein not only loved medical research but also loved being involved with patients; he was equally comfortable in the laboratory or on the hospital wards.[8] Hence, research that led to advances at the patient's bedside—what we now know as "translational research"—was what motivated him. It was certainly not the lure of money. He was not suited to business, clearly recounting a story from his youth in which he was the only one who managed to lose money investing in a "sure bet" carnival stand.[9] The standard issue, government laboratories with their metal, olive-drab file cabinets, and the fertile and focused research environment at WRAIR suited him.

Artenstein's research team for the meningococcal effort took shape by the fall of 1966, with the addition of two recently inducted physician scientists—Emil Gotschlich and Irving Goldschneider. Gotschlich had decided after his Bellevue Hospital internship that he preferred research to clinical medicine and had spent six subsequent years at the Rockefeller Institute in an immunochemistry lab; his path to meningococcal work was fairly direct—"I was drafted, simple as that".[10] Goldschneider had also been drafted straight out of medical school at the University of Pennsylvania but managed to elude entering active duty until he had completed his residency training in pathology at Case Western in Cleveland. By that time, he already had laboratory experience in immunology research; thus, the meningococcal vaccine project was a good fit.[11]

Now, with the right talent in place, the WRAIR group set about the task of solving the puzzle of how to protect susceptible individuals from acquiring meningococcal meningitis. The research was a high priority for the Army given the ongoing threats and realities of meningococcal outbreaks at basic training posts throughout the country. With the war in Vietnam escalating and exponentially increasing numbers of recruits pouring into these sites to prepare for deployments, Artenstein and his group were under steady pressure to make progress. Nonetheless, they took an organized, well-reasoned approach to the work; they knew no other way. In order to move the research along most efficiently, several interrelated lines of investigation were conducted concurrently.

Goldschneider took the lead on the studies to delineate human immune responses against the meningococcus. These experiments were designed to identify certain individuals who might be at risk of disease—the "susceptibles"—and whether there were those who were somehow naturally protected against getting sick—the "immune." If the researchers could identify people—in this case young Army recruits—who seemed to be protected from the infection, perhaps they could find a common link in their immune responses—something that they could try to artificially induce with a vaccine.

Gotschlich, who had come to WRAIR by way of the Rockefeller Institute, was therefore quite familiar with the four-decade-old work of Avery and Heidelberger there on the "specific soluble substance"—capsular polysaccharide—and its role in determining the immunologic specificity of pneumococci. Like Kabat, he would use his immunochemistry background to ascertain whether the capsular polysaccharide of the meningococcus possessed similar properties and could be used like bait—to attract the attention of the immune response and potentially serve as a vaccine. At least there was precedent for this concept; MacLeod and Heidelberger had shown it with a pneumococcal polysaccharide vaccine in troops at the Army Air Force Technical School in Sioux Falls twenty years earlier.

The lack of a suitable animal model that mimicked the route and course of infection in humans meant that the WRAIR group would need to work with human specimens for their immunology research on the meningococcus. And these were procured from a vast collection of bacterial cultures and blood samples from recruits with meningitis—anywhere in the Army—that Artenstein had arranged to be frozen and delivered to their laboratory. Additionally, knowing that one of the first events in basic training for every new military recruit was a complete physical examination—which included the collection of blood for routine lab testing— Artenstein managed to secure 15,000 of these blood samples collected from new recruits at Fort Dix, New Jersey, one of the busiest and largest training centers in the Army, in a five-month period during the winter of 1967–1968. The serum portion of these samples—saved in Artenstein's freezers at WRAIR—would come in handy to study when some of these recruits later developed meningococcal meningitis during basic training—an all-too frequent occurrence.

A number of observations from the 1940s—before the antimicrobial "miracle" drugs had caused researchers to move on to other problems—informed the work on meningococcal immunity. It was well known at the time that even during epidemics of meningococcal meningitis in military camps, most young recruits do not get sick with the infection. However, many carry the germ in their noses and throats— asymptomatically—for a period of time. It was also known that many diseases of childhood—such as measles and certain streptococcal infections—occurred only in kids with low levels of serum antibody against these pathogens. In fact measles vaccine, licensed just three years before the WRAIR group started their meningococcal vaccine research, worked by inducing the formation of just such antibodies.

Finally, attacks of meningococcal meningitis appeared to confer immunity against subsequent infections with the same strain of bacteria; this seemed to hold true in humans, and Kabat had shown this experimentally in mice. Many species of animal were known to have antibodies against meningococci in their blood under natural conditions, possibly explaining the difficulty in creating a suitable animal model that simulated meningitis in humans. Therefore, mounting evidence suggested that antibodies against meningococci were important in protection against infection, but definitive proof of this was lacking. The WRAIR research would provide this proof.

As it so happened that winter at Fort Dix, an outbreak of group C meningococcal infection occurred, causing sixty cases of systemic disease—an all too common phenomenon at recruit centers during the 1960s. Using the serum samples that Artenstein had collected from the arrival physical exams of soldiers at Fort Dix and the various meningococcal strains that he had acquired from around the world, Goldschneider measured antibodies directed against the polysaccharide capsule of meningococci—anticapsular antibodies. The results showed that more than eighty percent of the recruits—none of whom became infected—had preexisting antibody that killed the epidemic strain and other strains of the bacteria. However, only five percent of those who developed meningococcal disease had preexisting, bacterial-killing antibodies in their serum.[12]

It was clear from these experiments that anticapsular antibody circulating in the blood was responsible for protecting the recruits against systemic meningococcal disease during epidemics. But how did it get there? And why were there relatively few cases—sixty—of meningococcal disease even though a substantial number—almost 3,000—of recruits lacked antibody when they had their blood drawn during the first week of basic?

The answer became apparent when they studied another training company of recruits at Fort Dix in 1968. The WRAIR researchers found that eleven percent—fifty-four out of 492—of these men were susceptible to meningococcal disease by virtue of the absence of antibodies in their serum—they had never been exposed to it before the Army. However, during the eight-week course of basic training, more than ninety percent of those fifty-four recruits became asymptomatic carriers of the germ. In thirteen of these, the germ they carried was the same strain as the one that was causing the outbreak; nearly forty percent of those men became sick with meningococcal disease. Thus, there appeared to be a very high risk of meningococcal meningitis for people who were exposed to a dangerous strain of the bacteria for the first time.[12]

The carrier state, which occurred in most of the recruits who did not have serum antibody against meningococci upon arrival at basic training, served to immunize them—they developed serum antibody against the meningococcus just by harboring the organism in their throats—and therefore protected most of them from getting infected with the epidemic strain. Almost all became asymptomatic carriers early in the course of the eight-week basic training period, explaining the well-known observation that it was the newest recruits who were most vulnerable to meningococcal meningitis; seasoned troops were less susceptible to infection.[13]

Putting all the pieces together, the WRAIR investigators reasoned that the pathway of immunity to meningococcal infection proceeds like this: most young adults have been exposed over the course of their lives to various meningococci—usually passed along from the mouth and throat of someone else who is temporarily carrying the germ; the bacteria then transiently set up shop in their new hosts' throats, inducing the formation of antibodies against the polysaccharide capsule which circulate in their blood. These antibodies have long memories, respond rapidly when needed, and last for many years—and it is these antibodies that protect them against meningococcal disease.

Over time, the same process occurs with different strains of meningococci, expanding the breadth of their immune protection. However, occasionally—especially when a dangerous, epidemic strain is circulating in the environment—meningococci may be passed to the throats of young people who have not been exposed before. When this happens, that individual is at high risk of developing meningococcal meningitis. How can this be prevented? The hypothesis of the WRAIR group was that by priming the immune system of new recruits with a polysaccharide vaccine, they could artificially—in the absence of an actual bacterial infection—induce a state of protective immunity against the strain in the vaccine.

The reason that meningococcal epidemics tended to occur frequently in military recruit camps is that there, large groups of young men of different immunologic exposure backgrounds were gathered together into what was essentially a large germ incubator. In this enclosed environment where young potential hosts were intimately exposed to one another for long periods of time—training, eating, defecating, sleeping, coughing, and breathing—infectious agents were easily passed around. Meningococci, like many of these agents, are transmitted via respiratory secretions; coughing, sneezing, or even just breathing in close proximity to others could expose them to the germ. In this large collection of young men, many would already have serum antibody against meningococci, and some would be unwittingly carrying various meningococci in their throats at the time. However, others—a minority as we have seen—would be "susceptible" to meningococcal infection. And a significant proportion of this relatively small number of individuals would develop systemic meningococcal disease. Because of the massive troop numbers, it was almost predictable that some of these recruits would come down with meningococcal disease under these circumstances—and some would die.

With a clear understanding of the protective immune response to meningococcal meningitis—strain-specific, serum antibody against the polysaccharide capsule— the WRAIR group embarked on efforts to produce a version of the polysaccharide coat that would effectively provoke the desired response. By invoking some novel immunochemistry techniques, Gotschlich succeeded in doing what Kabat was unable to do two decades earlier—he prepared high molecular weight, purified, groups A and C meningococcal polysaccharides[14] that were highly immunogenic— capable of artificially inducing a strong antibody response—in humans.[15] Gotschlich proved this by testing the material on himself. Then, five additional human volunteers, including Artenstein and Goldschneider, were injected with the polysaccharides—once the material was shown not to cause fevers or significant weight loss in mice and guinea pigs. They had their blood drawn and their throats cultured multiple times afterwards; all showed excellent anticapsular antibody responses.

The decision to act as "guinea pigs" for their own vaccine was an easy one; there is a long and storied tradition of such self-experimentation in medical research.[16] As we have seen, Jenner's mentor, John Hunter, was reported to have contracted both gonorrhea and syphilis—intentionally in the case of the former and inadvertently with the latter—from the practice. Walter Reed—the namesake of WRAIR—was the only member of his team in Cuba not to have exposed himself to yellow fever-infected mosquitoes in an attempt to prove the insect's role in transmission of the virus; other team members died in the effort.

In vaccine research, it was almost expected that the investigators would be the first to sample their own products, both as a show of faith in their science and also so they could accurately report—first-hand—on its side effects, especially when they subsequently went to recruit study volunteers. For the WRAIR investigators, self-experimentation—even on their children—was second nature. However, this was an Army facility and five of the six original volunteers were on active duty. Their commanding officer did not like the idea that they might be jeopardizing military property—themselves—but tacitly complied.

If their crude vaccine could prevent throat carriage also, it would theoretically prevent the transmission of pathogenic meningococci from one individual to another, which would go a long way towards aborting the spread of a meningococcal epidemic. Artenstein and the group headed back to Fort Dix in early 1968 to prove this and were able to recruit 145 newly arrived, yet cold and tired recruits who volunteered to get injected with the group C meningococcal polysaccharide vaccine. When asked, all that they could tell the soldiers about its safety was that the researchers had injected themselves and had not experienced any serious side effects.[9] Six weeks later, they had their proof; significantly fewer men who received the vaccine had become carriers of the group C meningococcus as compared with those who did not receive it.[17]

Gotschlich and Goldschneider returned to civilian life in the summer of 1968; Gotschlich went back to the Rockefeller, where he would spend the rest of his career, and Goldschneider became an immunology researcher at the University of Connecticut. Both, as we shall soon see, continued their meningococcal work. Artenstein—armed with an understanding of the immunologic "correlate of protection"—anticapsular antibody—of meningococcal infection and some limited information on the safety of the home-grown polysaccharide vaccine and its ability to provoke such an antibody response in humans, decided it was time to find out if their vaccine worked under actual "field" conditions. The Army command—embattled by both the deleterious impact on the "fighting strength" and the bad public relations engendered by ongoing meningococcal outbreaks at basic training sites—gave the go-ahead.

To do so would require a large-scale, clinical vaccine trial—a logistical nightmare—given what the WRAIR investigators knew about the epidemiology of meningococcal disease in the Army. These studies would have to be executed at basic training sites, where the risk of infection was highest. However, because there were few cases relative to the entire group of recruits at any one location—even during outbreaks—and because of the unpredictable occurrence of meningococcal disease—even during epidemics—a number of the largest, busiest, military recruit embarkation centers would need to be involved, enrolling study volunteers simultaneously. This was the only way to rapidly accrue an adequate sample size—the number of subjects under study—to determine if the vaccine truly prevented meningococcal disease.

In clinical research, statistics are of paramount importance; they are used to compare one group—in this case the vaccinated group—against another group—the unvaccinated, "control" group. In order for the results of a study to be valid, there must be enough members of each group and enough possible outcomes—cases of meningococcal meningitis—for the statistics to conclude that any differences between the two groups were related to the vaccine and not to random chance—coincidence. Hence, it was critical to enroll enough soldiers to answer the question definitively—does the vaccine prevent meningitis?

Why was it important to enroll the study so swiftly? Artenstein had learned from their basic research that only the new recruits were vulnerable; after the first weeks of basic training, the troops became less susceptible to meningococcal infection, as they were exposed to various strains, became temporary carriers, and developed immunity on this basis. Therefore, he had to design the trial so that informed consent—an Army regulation and the right thing to do for any experimental product—and vaccination of new recruits would be completed within days of the men arriving at basic training.

Basic training in the Army was a protocol-driven, eight-week exercise that had been honed to near science—through decades of experience—by the time of the Vietnam War. There, in grueling sixteen hours training days, new military recruits—most of them draftees—were taught the fundamental skills needed for combat; they were also subjected to large doses of psychological manipulation, designed to make them behave as a unit, rather than as a group of individuals.[18-20] During the 1960s, as American involvement in combat progressively escalated and with it the need for fresh troops, recruits arrived with regularity and around the clock to the Army's large recruit training centers, brought by bus from their hometowns around the country. At Fort Dix, for instance, as many as 15,000 new recruits might arrive weekly, joining the thousands of other trainees already there in a continuous flow of troop movement.

Upon arrival, new recruits were part of "reception battalion"—the week or so period before training actually began in which the men were "processed"—given haircuts; completed paperwork; issued uniforms; underwent physical examinations, mandatory vaccinations, and dental checkups; received instruction in marching and military bearing; and took a physical assessment test. At the end of this period, groups of recruits—"training units"—were picked up by their drill sergeants and marched off to their barracks—their homes for the first two months of their new lives as soldiers. The same process was repeated weekly for dozens of thousands of recruits at multiple sites throughout the U.S.

For Artenstein and his trial teams at each facility, that week before boot camp actually began was their window of opportunity to gather groups of recruits, explain their study, answer all questions, obtain permission from the volunteers, randomly assign them to either receive the vaccine or to be in the control group, and vaccinate those who were chosen. Then, the recruits were given the other required vaccines—influenza, polio, and tetanus toxoid—along with the rest of their platoon. All of this was to be accomplished within days of their arrival at the training center—a particularly impressive feat given that many of these recruits were often tired, scared, and away from home for the first time in their young lives. But they were more scared by the prospect of becoming sick with meningitis, which made recruitment slightly easier.

The first, large, vaccine field trial began in late January 1969 and involved 13,763 recruits immunized with a group C meningococcal polysaccharide vaccine at five of the Army's largest basic training centers: Fort Dix, New Jersey; Fort Polk, Louisiana; Fort Knox, Kentucky, site of the Army's 1st Armored—tank—Division; Fort Bragg, North Carolina, home to the Airborne and Special Forces; and Fort Lewis, Washington.[21] A second trial, beginning in the spring of 1969 and lasting through early 1970, involved 14,482 soldiers who were vaccinated at three large recruit centers.[22] It was an enormous undertaking. In addition to the more than 28,000 men who received the experimental vaccine, nearly 115,000 recruits served as unvaccinated controls. Study teams at each of the sites coordinated the activities on the ground; Artenstein and his WRAIR team directed the whole project, making frequent trips to each field location.

When the dust had settled, both trials gave almost identical results. In each, only one case of meningococcal disease due to group C—the strain contained in the vaccine—was identified in the vaccinated men, and one of those cases was diagnosed just 9 days after vaccination—probably insufficient time to elicit an immune response. In contrast, 73 cases of group C meningococcal meningitis occurred among the recruits who had not received vaccine. The vaccine was found to be safe, with only minimal redness or tenderness—expected side effects—at the injection site in some recruits.

The final verdict on the vaccine—it was effective; its use resulted in a nearly ninety percent reduction in cases of meningitis caused by group C meningococci. Almost immediately—based on these dramatic findings—the Army gave the go-ahead for the WRAIR group to arrange for large-scale, commercial manufacture of the vaccine, leading to the first widespread deployment of an effective polysaccharide vaccine. Within 18 months of the completion of these efficacy trials, the routine use of group C meningococcal polysaccharide vaccine to protect against meningococcal disease at basic training centers virtually eliminated this pathogen as a health problem in the military.[23]

Within a decade, using the concepts derived from the WRAIR group—ideas that were themselves derived from the work of Avery, Heidelberger, Kabat, MacLeod, and others—a polysaccharide vaccine containing four meningococcal groups—a "quadrivalent" vaccine—was given to all military recruits when they arrived at basic training. In this fashion, outbreaks of meningococcal disease within the military—caused by the strains represented in the vaccine—no longer presented a problem.

Artenstein would not be a part of this chapter of the work; he died in 1976—at the age of 46—of liver failure caused by laboratory-acquired hepatitis, just five years after the triumphant success of the first meningococcal polysaccharide vaccine. But he had lived to witness the fruits of his labors remove the specter of epidemic meningococcal meningitis as a threat to troops.

The same, quadrivalent, polysaccharide vaccine approach was also used to prevent sporadic cases of meningococcal disease in those at risk, such as college students living in dormitories and people traveling to regions known to harbor epidemic disease. However, shortly after the book was closed on the first, effective meningococcal polysaccharide vaccine, events elsewhere in the world would shine a light on the need for better, broader, more effective vaccines to protect those who were traditionally at the highest risk of meningococcal meningitis—children.

Chapter 10
Success for Half

When Dr. Martin Randolph came to Danbury, a small city in the southwestern corner of Connecticut, in 1948, the medical establishment there was ill prepared for this young, energetic, academic pediatrician. In this former "hat city"—so named because a large proportion of America's hats were made there in the early twentieth century—general practitioners practiced everything from pediatrics to surgery. Randolph was a different breed—the first board certified pediatrician in Danbury—who continued his research on new treatments and vaccines while maintaining a busy private practice out of his home office.[1]

Randolph successfully advocated for the widespread adoption of the new vaccines—as they became available in the 1950s and 1960s—against polio, measles, and mumps in children. By the early 1970s, he was the health advisor to the public and parochial schools and in this capacity, through his academic ties to nearby Yale and with the backing of his brother-in-law—the city's director of health, he was able to attract research studies to Danbury.[2]

Fresh off the success of the meningococcal vaccine work at WRAIR, Goldschneider—now a civilian—had relocated to the University of Connecticut Medical Center, a monolithic structure arising from a hilltop on the 106-acre O'Meara farm tract in suburban Hartford that had opened its doors shortly before he arrived. There, he met Martha Lepow, a pediatric infectious diseases researcher with a track record in vaccine studies. Together, they decided "it was time to take meningococcal A and C vaccines to the kids".[3]

Lepow possessed a vaccine researcher's pedigree. After graduating from medical school in 1952, she had studied viruses in the laboratory of Fred Robbins at Case Western in Cleveland. Robbins, as we saw, shared the 1954 Nobel Prize with Enders and Weller for their landmark work in growing polioviruses in tissue culture—research that led directly to an effective vaccine against polio. Lepow became enamored with laboratory research there, deciding to make it a major part of her career. With her husband, who was recruited to be the Chair of Pathology, she joined the fledgling University of Connecticut Medical Center in 1967, launching the discipline of pediatric infectious diseases there and initiating a decade-long effort to advance the health of children by focusing on disease prevention using vaccines. Moving to Albany Medical School in 1978, she continued that mission—as she does there today—at the age of 85.

Goldschneider's original work at WRAIR on the natural course of immunity to the meningococcus in humans had shown that the most vulnerable period for the development of meningococcal meningitis was in young children between the ages of six months and two years; after that, there was a progressive decline in the number of cases except for a small blip in the rate that occurred in the young adult years—coincident with military service.[4] What the WRAIR investigators found most interesting, though, was the inverse—opposite—relationship between levels of serum antibody directed against the polysaccharide capsule and the number of meningitis cases; as the levels of antibody progressively rose, beginning in two-year-olds, the occurrence of disease rapidly decreased. As we have seen, by the late teens, most people had developed immunity to at least some strains of the meningo-coccus. By that time, those lacking immunity against an epidemic strain were at high risk of getting meningococcal meningitis in basic training or a similar setting.

Given this pattern, meningococcal infection appeared to behave similarly to other classic infections of childhood. Even before the availability of vaccinations for measles, polio, and diphtheria, all of these infections were known to be significantly more common at young ages. Case rates of these diseases, extremely low during the first six months of life, increased during early childhood and then began to decline after two years of age—around the same time that many children developed antibodies in their blood—through natural exposures or actual illness—to ward off the germ. Thus, naturally acquired antibody, even without clinical manifestations of disease, appeared to prevent infection against these pathogens. In fact, a twist on this concept—provoking the formation of protective antibodies by challenging children with weakened versions or proteins of a germ—was harnessed to create successful vaccines against these childhood scourges.

Why were there so few cases of the classic diseases of childhood or meningococcal meningitis during the first six months of life? That answer had begun to be understood shortly before the WRAIR group began their initial investigations. Neonates—newborn babies—have essentially no ability to generate their own immune responses against a world filled with potential, dangerous infectious threats. Fortunately though, they are the recipients of a final gift from their mothers before birth; antibodies from her blood are transferred through the placenta to the fetus. These represent a sampling from the mother's entire repertoire of antibodies against various infections—generated by numerous exposures or actual infections over the course of her lifetime—that can now be used to protect her newborn from these same problems. But the catch is they only persist for about six months; after that, the child must either make their own anti-body upon exposure to a particular germ or be artificially exposed by virtue of vacci-nation. The inherent downside of natural exposure to these pathogens, of course, is that it will sometimes result in severe illness.

Armed with an understanding of the process of immunity to meningococci gleaned from the WRAIR studies, Lepow and Goldschneider developed plans for vaccine trials in children. With group C and group A meningococcal vaccines provided by the Army via their contracted manufacturer—E.R. Squibb—they performed two, small pilot studies.

Twenty-two children of University of Connecticut faculty members, including Lepow's two sons and Goldschneider's eldest one, were administered group A meningococcal vaccine, which had already been tested in 600 military recruits and was found to be safe and capable of inducing antibodies against the bacteria.[5] The Army had not performed a large-scale clinical trial with this vaccine—as they had with group C vaccine—because there were too few cases of natural group A meningitis in the recruit camps to be able to measure whether the vaccine was protective. Twenty-six children, residents of nearby Newington Children's Hospital who ranged in age from seven months to nine years and had parental consent, were vaccinated with the group C vaccine. At Newington, a facility specializing in the care of children with chronic orthopedic and neurologic disabilities resulting from conditions such as Legg–Perthes disease, a congenital hip deformity; scoliosis, an abnormal curvature of the backbone; and various abnormalities of the spinal cord, the pediatric recipients could be closely monitored by the medical staff.[6] The results—the vaccine was safe from serious side effects and provoked an appropriate antibody response in the kids—were encouraging to the investigators, prompting a larger study.

The next step was to study the vaccine in younger children on a larger scale to determine its potential effectiveness in a pediatric population—of vital importance because of the high risk of disease in this group. They got permission to test the Army vaccine, and through Goldschneider's connections, they were able to obtain a supply—then only available to the military.[5] Using the successful model employed by Jonas Salk, who had executed the massive, national polio vaccine trial in elementary schools nearly two decades earlier, Lepow initially approached the West Hartford school superintendent in early 1972 and proposed to study first and second graders in the district where her children attended school.[3] She was rebuffed on the basis that "we do not do research in our schools." Undeterred, they would not have to look much farther afield to find their trial site.

Randolph, still actively engaged in academic medicine while juggling a busy, 100-hours per week solo pediatric practice, was in the audience in the early part of 1972 to hear Goldschneider and Lepow give a presentation on meningococcal vaccine research at Yale's pediatric grand rounds. In it they described their desire to perform a large clinical trial to study the effectiveness of the meningococcal A and C vaccines in young children. Afterwards, Randolph—the health advisor to Danbury's schools—approached the speakers with a proposal; he thought that he could arrange for them to perform the trial in Danbury because there, "the schools, the parents and the city in general, knew of the benefits from medical research and had become accustomed to trials of new vaccines".[2] To his everlasting credit, he made it happen.

In October 1972, in front of television cameras and their parents, 1,300 first and second graders from Danbury's eight public and four parochial schools who were bussed in to the north side of town—Hayestown Avenue elementary school—from all over the city, each received an injection in their arms.[2] In what represented the first, civilian, large-scale vaccination against meningitis in the U.S., the children received either the group A polysaccharide vaccine, group C vaccine, or no vaccine—the controls. Although the logistics were challenging—the kids were dressed against winter, necessitating removal and haphazard inventory of coats, sweaters, and mittens to get to their bare arms, all while additional busloads of children crowded into the school gymnasium—the study confirmed that school-age children generally responded well to the vaccines, making protective levels of antibodies that were directed against the bacteria.

Danbury represented the first large-scale evidence that the meningitis vaccines could be effective in children. For children—a historically large population of otherwise potential victims of meningococcal meningitis—the good news arrived none too soon; the information gleaned from these vaccine studies in the U.S. would—in short order—be put to the test under the extreme conditions of epidemic meningitis. Because around the time that healthy, first graders were being used as test subjects in a crowded elementary school gymnasium in southwest Connecticut, a year-old epidemic of sulfa drug-resistant, group C meningococcal meningitis was peaking nearly 5,000 miles to the south.

In the early 1970s, Saõ Paulo—with its population of more than eight million people—was Brazil's largest and most rapidly growing metropolitan area. The city was no stranger to epidemic meningococcal disease; twenty-five years earlier, the disease had struck and smoldered at outbreak levels for more than five years. Then—for unclear reasons—it receded, and only occasional, sporadic cases occurred for the next two decades. But in the spring of 1971, health authorities there noticed an abrupt spike in the numbers of cases of meningococcal disease—reaching epidemic levels and staying there—even rising—for the next eighteen months.[7] The authorities were able to obtain accurate case counts because it was required that all suspect cases of meningitis be sent to the Hospital Emilio Ribas—the city's "isolation hospital" when it opened a century earlier—the main public health care facility in Saõ Paulo.

During the prolonged epidemic in Saõ Paulo, there were more than 2,000 total cases of meningococcal disease; nearly ten percent of its victims died, despite the availability of multiple different antibiotic drug treatments. Infants—children below the age of one year—and kids up to age two were disproportionately affected; they suffered both the highest attack rates and the highest fatality rates—more than forty percent of all the deaths were in this group—among all of those sick with meningococcal disease.

Brazilian health authorities, needing some intervention to quell the burgeoning outbreak in their largest city and aware of the success of group C meningococcal polysaccharide vaccine in the U.S. military, sought help. Based on the successful results of hundreds of thousands of recruits who had received the vaccine over the preceding two years and the recent, small-scale information on the apparent effectiveness—at least in promoting useful antibody responses—of the vaccine in children from the University of Connecticut studies, the U.S. government approved the deployment of vaccine to Saõ Paulo. In a ten-day period just before Christmas of 1972, 67,000 children between the ages of six months and three years were vaccinated. What became clear from this effort was that the vaccine proved effective in children more than two years old—subsequently preventing thousands of cases and hundreds of deaths due to meningococcal meningitis in Brazil—yet it failed to protect the youngest children.[8]

In other field trials in the early 1970s, meningococcal polysaccharide vaccines proved their mettle in preventing cases of meningitis or stopping the spread of out-breaks of disease. In Sudan[9]—part of the African "meningitis belt," where epidemic meningitis occurred regularly—and in Egypt[10]—where disease was ever present—group A vaccine in civilian young adults and school children showed strikingly similar—and favorable—results to those of the WRAIR studies in Army recruits. As with group C vaccine in the U.S. Army, group A meningococcal vaccine was shown to be highly protective—nearly ninety percent—in preventing meningitis during an outbreak among military recruits in Finland.[11] Therefore, by the mid-1970s, there was a general sense that meningococcal polysaccharide vaccines were highly useful to prevent meningococcal meningitis in children and adults and could even be used to halt the spread of epidemics. However, there was still the sticky, yet critical, issue of protecting those who most needed protection from meningococcal disease—infants and toddlers.

Problems with vaccine-induced protective immunity in the six month to two-year-old age group were not a new issue; this age-related phenomenon had been observed with certain other childhood vaccines. During the first six months of life—but most significantly in the first three months—infants use antibodies donated by their mothers to protect them against infectious diseases, as we have previously seen. Between months three and six of age and certainly after that, they must go it alone—generating their own immune responses against would-be invaders like bacteria and viruses in order to protect themselves. The dilemma is that early on their immune systems are on a very steep learning curve at the same time they are engaged in this fight for survival against infectious threats. And the process of mounting an immune response after vaccination with polysaccharides appeared to be too advanced a lesson for these immature immune systems.

A part of the Danbury studies had involved vaccinating infants—some as young as ten weeks of age—with meningococcal polysaccharides. Some of these children were patients from Dr. Randolph's large pediatric practice. In general, these experiments confirmed what had been seen in the field use of the vaccine: kids under two years of age made significantly lower antibody responses than older children to the vaccine; the vaccine was more effective with every passing month of life after the first three but still failed to reach protective levels; and the number of injections did not seem to influence the responses.[12] The bottom line was that infants—the ones with the greatest vulnerability to meningococcal disease and death—were the least likely to benefit from the vaccines. Something would need to be done to enhance the effect of the meningococcal polysaccharides. That "something" would emerge from research over the next decade—research that had its origins in sixty-year-old work out of the Rockefeller Institute by a future Nobel laureate and the "Professor"—Oswald Avery.

Karl Landsteiner—already at the ripe old age of 55 when he began working at the Rockefeller Institute for Medical Research in 1922—had forged a distinguished career in science in his native Vienna for a quarter of a century before heading to New York. After completing medical school at the University of Vienna, he studied chemistry, bacteriology, and pathology, subsequently serving as an assistant to Professor Anton Weichselbaum—the discoverer of the bacterial cause of epidemic cerebrospinal meningitis—at the Pathological Institute there for twelve years.[13] Thus, in another example of "six degrees of separation," Landsteiner's ultimate, albeit indirect, contribution to meningococcal vaccines had direct connections to the origins of the disease itself.

Working under Weichselbaum in the first years of the twentieth century, Landsteiner began the landmark work that would lead to his discovery of human blood groups—earning him the Nobel Prize in Medicine or Physiology thirty years later for that accomplishment. In 1908, while still in Vienna, he became the first to experimentally transmit polio from human tissue to animals—nonhuman primates— and in so doing, reproduce the disease in that species. Hence, Landsteiner was already an internationally renowned scientist by the time he began the next phase of his career at Rockefeller.

In the decade preceding his arrival in New York, Landsteiner—examining the chemistry of antibodies—had discovered that certain substances did not stimulate the production of antibodies when injected into animals; they could only provoke a specific antibody response if they were attached to a protein.[14] The antibodies subsequently elicited were targeted against both components of the combination. He hypothesized that the protein in this situation acted as both a carrier of the second substance and a facilitator—orchestrating and promoting antibody formation.

Landsteiner's work undoubtedly influenced one of his new colleagues at Rockefeller—Oswald Avery. "Fess"—short for "the Professor"—as Avery was affectionately known there, had already shown with Heidelberger that the "specific soluble substance"—a polysaccharide—was both the inducer and the target of immunity in pneumococcal infection. In the late 1920s, Avery used Landsteiner's theory to prove that linking—"conjugating"—polysaccharide to proteins could enhance the antibody response to these complex sugars.[15] A half a century later, two research teams—one at Children's Hospital Boston and another from the National Institutes of Health—succeeded in applying Landsteiner's and Avery's concept of conjugation to improve the strength and the duration of antibody responses to another important cause of sporadic cases of meningitis in very young children— Hemophilus influenzae type b—Hib.

The bacteria Hib, like the meningococcus and pneumococcus, also had a polysaccharide capsule and as with these germs, antibody directed against this sugar coating conferred immunity. However, as with many such organisms, this immunity was age related. The most vulnerable group—infants and the very young—were the same ones that had both the least intrinsic ability to protect themselves and the lowest capability to develop an immune response to injected polysaccharide vaccines. The researchers solved this puzzle by attaching the Hib polysaccharide to diphtheria toxoid proteins—the ones used in the effective, childhood, diphtheria vaccine.[16] This conjugate vaccine proved to be highly effective in preventing Hib disease in infants as young as two months of age. It entered into routine clinical use in pediatrics in the early 1990s, virtually eliminating Hib meningitis—previously a major cause of disease among young children—as a medical problem in the developed world.

How do conjugate vaccines—linking the polysaccharide of interest to a carrier protein—manage to provoke strong, long-lasting antibodies in infants when the polysaccharides themselves cannot? The answer lies in the fundamental operations of the immune system. Short of developing and recovering from an infection—a risky proposition in many cases—vaccines represent the best way to induce a state of immunity against a particular germ. As we have seen earlier, there are multiple different types of vaccines. The vaccines effective in preventing meningococcal disease in children and young adults are composed of the polysaccharide subunit of various strains of these bacteria. But as we have also seen, the polysaccharides themselves are not sufficient to provoke a strong, effective, and long-lasting state of immunity in infants and very young kids. The main reason for this appears to be that these vaccines only activate one of the two main "arms" of the human immune response, and those with the most immature immune systems—children below the age of two—need both arms to be working together in order to generate an effective antibody response against a polysaccharide.

Unlike polysaccharides, vaccines made from proteins such as diphtheria or tetanus toxoids; measles, mumps, or rubella, which comprise weakened versions of live viruses; or influenza or the Salk polio vaccines, which are composed of killed germs, stimulate both arms of the immune system. This allows protein-based vaccines—and germs are largely made of proteins—to maximally provoke the formation of strong antibody responses directed against the material in the vaccine. By chemically joining a bacterial polysaccharide with a specific protein molecule, the full spectrum of the immune response can be stimulated, promoting the development of high, effective, and durable levels of antibodies that can be rekindled—"boosted"—by subsequent doses of vaccine when they fall below protective levels.

By employing the concept of conjugation over the past fifteen years, new meningococcal vaccines have dramatically impacted the burden of disease and its mortality—especially in young children—in the parts of the world where these vaccines are routinely used. They continue to be improved upon—usually by either changing the protein carrier molecule or broadening the meningococcal polysaccharides to include multiple, different strains—and studied in clinical trials. The introduction and childhood use of polysaccharide–protein conjugate vaccines against other bacteria, most notably that more than century-old scourge—the pneumococcus—have led to dramatic reductions in severe, invasive pneumococcal disease in high-risk individuals, and a significant lowering of the economic burden of middle ear infections in children due to this bacterium. An additional windfall from the reduced overall impact of pneumococcal infections with the use of conjugated vaccines in childhood has been a major reduction in the rate of antibiotic-resistant strains—a tremendous benefit to society.[17]

The past 40 years—beginning with the work at WRAIR and continuing through the development of effective meningococcal conjugate vaccines—have witnessed tremendous advances in the prevention and control of meningococcal meningitis. In the U.S., Western Europe, and other portions of the developed world, this has translated into fewer sporadic cases of disease among those at risk and the ability to stave off outbreaks when the conditions are ripe for these. But despite the successes and reason for continued optimism as vaccines against many types of meningococci continue to evolve, there remain major gaps in the control of this disease.

In parts of the developing world, especially in the "meningitis belt" extending across sub-Saharan Africa and in areas of Russia and Asia as well, periodic and recurrent epidemics of meningococcal meningitis continue to decimate and devastate the population. As is the case with the control or prevention of other acute and chronic infectious diseases in resource-starved areas, the problem often boils down to economic imperatives; vaccines against meningococci, although available, have not been deployed due to financial, political, and logistical constraints. A strategy is in place to potentially address much of this in Africa, as we shall soon see. However, another type of meningococcal disease—that due to group B meningococci—has eluded a vaccine solution for entirely different reasons, and it continues to represent an important shortcoming in the prevention of this disease.

Group B meningococcus accounts for a significant burden of sporadic cases of meningitis in the U.S. and elsewhere in the developed world. There, like many other germs, it is "endemic"—maintained in the infectious landscape as a continual cause of disease without the need to introduce it from elsewhere. Group B accounts for approximately half of the cases of meningococcal disease in the United States and an even higher proportion in Europe, where it has displaced other, vaccine-preventable, meningococcal groups.[18] It also causes a high burden of meningitis in infants and has caused outbreaks of the disease around the world. But even if the use of the most effective, currently available meningococcal vaccines were expanded globally, these problems would not be solved because group B is not one of the types included in current vaccines.

The dilemma with the polysaccharide capsule of group B meningococci is that it does not provoke an antibody response in humans, as do the polysaccharides of groups A and C for instance. This was observed early on in small-scale studies performed by Artenstein's group at WRAIR using the same methods to prepare vaccine that had been employed for their successful studies with other meningococcal groups.[19] Why does the sugar-coated exterior of this strain of bacteria behave differently than that of the other meningococci? Although the answer to this quandary has been largely elucidated, a vaccine solution remains to be seen.

Biochemical and immunologic differences between the polysaccharide capsules of groups B and C meningococci had been categorized by the WRAIR group and were further described by Gotschlich upon his return to the Rockefeller Institute in the late 1960s. The exterior coat of group B meningococci contains structures with certain biochemical properties that mirror those found in some of the most commonly occurring bacteria—*Escherichia coli*—that are normal colonizers of the human intestines.[20] Additionally, group B meningococci extend this practice of "molecular mimicry" to other components of human tissues; certain molecules within the human brain and nervous system—like certain normal intestinal bacteria—share biochemical and structural properties with the bacteria's polysaccharide capsule.[21] This explains why group B polysaccharide vaccines—the same preparations that proved to be so successful in preventing meningococcal disease caused by groups A and C bacteria in military recruits—failed to evoke protective antibody responses.

The human immune system is an intricate, well-coordinated, nimble, and highly 'matrixed' structure that is organized to respond rapidly—and with deadly force—to external threats to the body from entities such as bacteria, viruses, parasites, and noxious toxins. It is also programmed to survey and manage certain internal threats, such as the transformation of normal cells to become tumor cells, an early step in the development of cancers. A key caveat of this complex orchestration of defenses is that it must—and does—recognize our own cells, tissues, and other human structures as "self" and therefore does not target these for destruction. To do so, would lead to immunologic anarchy—widespread tissue breakdown—as occurs in some "autoimmune" disease states such as lupus or rheumatoid arthritis.

Thus, the human immune system rigorously—unless reprogrammed by some system glitch—practices a policy of strict "tolerance," leaving be those structures that it views as belonging to its human host. Group B meningococci—like some other pathogens—use this otherwise laudable attribute against their host, as a mechanism to evade the immune system and go about their dangerous business.[22] The ultimate control and prevention of group B meningococcal disease, like that caused by various epidemic strains of meningococci around the world, will require creative approaches that either address the scientific issues—as with group B—or the practical ones, so dominant with vaccine strategies in the developing world.

Chapter 11
The Future of a Killer

The first, documented one hundred years of cerebrospinal meningitis, during which the clinical course and worldwide occurrence of diseases were vividly described, was dominated by attempts at symptomatic and "alexipharmic"—antidote—therapy. That approach did little to alter the natural course and invariably fatal conclusion to this devastating disease. By the time that the clinical entity—now understood to be meningococcal meningitis—entered its second century, the body of knowledge in the sister sciences of microbiology and immunology had evolved to such a degree that it could support rigorous laboratory and clinical investigations of infectious diseases. This led to research—initially and largely carried out in the Institutes of the great cities of Europe—Paris, Vienna, and Berlin—but later advanced in New York, resulting in the first effective therapy for meningococcal disease. By 1907, the mortality rate would drop from seventy-five percent to thirty percent; physicians and scientists around the world felt as if they now had some measure of control against the infection.

Beginning in the 1930s with the discovery of the first, specific antibacterial drugs and continuing on for the next few decades, these "miracle" cures—antibiotics—further reduced the death rate of meningococcal disease, down to ten percent. In fact, antibacterial drugs were capable of preventing the disease in the first place if given before the initial signs or symptoms. Physicians became complacent; there was a sense that infectious diseases—up until that time among the most common and gravest threats to life and limb—could be forever vanquished as a cause for concern. However, within just a few years of the widespread use of these treatments, it had become clear that they were not the panacea initially envisioned.

With every new antibacterial drug introduced—and there were many during the mid-twentieth century—bacterial pathogens demonstrated new ways to rapidly become resistant to their beneficial effects. Outbreaks of antibiotic-resistant meningococcal meningitis occurred with increasing frequency during that time, most notably not only around military recruit camps but also in civilian populations around the world. As America prepared for war once again in the 1960s, it became clear that vaccines to prevent disease were the best hope for the eventual control of meningococcal meningitis. The invention of the first, effective polysaccharide

A.W. Artenstein, *In the Blink of an Eye: The Deadly Story of Epidemic Meningitis*, DOI 10.1007/978-1-4614-4845-7_11, © Springer Science+Business Media New York 2013

vaccine against these germs demonstrated the path to this goal; the evolution of meningococcal vaccines over the past four decades has illuminated it.

After two centuries of epidemic meningococcal meningitis, there are now multiple, effective vaccine solutions, yet several residual, vexing problems regarding this disease remain unresolved. A polysaccharide vaccine that combines preparations of the capsules from four of the most common serogroups—a "quadrivalent" vaccine—has been used since the early 1980s. This first-generation vaccine combines polysaccharides from the four types of meningococci that are most commonly responsible for sporadic and epidemic disease—groups A and C, and two other groups found in various parts of the world—Y and W-135. It has been used largely in developed countries for prevention of disease in those at risk such as military recruits, college students living in dormitories, patients with deficiencies of their immune systems, or travelers to areas experiencing meningitis epidemics. The vaccine is not effective and therefore not recommended for use in children below the age of two years, as we have seen previously, although children as young as three months of age may demonstrate a short-term benefit of the vaccine, which makes it potentially useful in temporarily containing outbreaks.

The most commonly occurring meningococcal serogroups in the Americas and Europe are B, C, and increasingly, Y.[1] Group B, not included in any of the currently available vaccines, now causes a majority of disease in many parts of the world; to some extent, it has filled in and replaced other groups that are covered in the vaccine. Group A meningococci—now rarely seen in the developed world—are the major causes of recurring, devastating epidemics in Africa, China, and elsewhere in the developing world. Other serogroups such as C, W-135, and the relatively uncommon, group X, also contribute—albeit to much lesser degrees—to the meningitis problem there.

Because of the poor activity of polysaccharide vaccines in very young children—a major shortcoming that was successfully dealt with by linking polysaccharides to protein carriers—"conjugate" vaccines for meningococcal disease first became available for use in the late 1990s. The deployment of a group C meningococcal conjugate vaccine, comprising polysaccharide linked to either tetanus or diphtheria proteins, among preschool and school-aged children in the UK in 1999 proved highly effective, reducing meningitis cases and deaths by more than ninety percent. The vaccine even resulted in substantially lower numbers of meningococcal carriers among people who were not vaccinated—"herd" immunity. Therefore, the population in general benefitted from fewer meningococci circulating in the environment and the lower numbers of individuals with meningitis who could potentially transmit infection.[2]

A quadrivalent conjugate vaccine—containing the same meningococcal groups as in the older, first-generation quadrivalent vaccine but now linked to diphtheria toxoid—was licensed in the U.S. in 2005.[3] Based on studies comparing its ability to provoke potentially protective antibody responses with those of the older polysaccharide vaccine, the meningococcal conjugate vaccine has been recommended as a routine immunization for adolescents and as an optional one for all children and adults—up to age 55—at increased risk of meningococcal disease. This particular conjugate vaccine has relatively poor activity in infants, prompting expanded development of more promising conjugates in the future for this population of potential meningitis victims.

Thus, the fundamental tools—conjugate vaccines against multiple serogroups—appear to be in place to embark on the final push towards prevention and control of meningococcal disease. But there remain significant impediments to realizing this ultimate goal. A major cause of worldwide disease—group B meningococcus—currently eludes a vaccine solution, for the reasons we have previously seen; in the African "meningitis belt," frequent, cyclic, and sometimes massive, recurrent epidemics of meningococcal disease continue to devastate the overwhelmingly young population there. How will these problems be addressed? Which direction will future control take?

The approach to each of these two dilemmas currently hindering the prevention and control of meningococcal disease around the world has been distinct. Addressing the problem of group B meningococcal meningitis, by necessity, has required innovative strategies derived from the biology of the organism—in some cases using molecular-based methods that were not even in the realm of possibility just a decade ago. Here, the issue is one of designing a vaccine that can induce protective immunity directed against a germ that appears to the human immune system—from the outside at least—like part of its own human host. Conversely, the problem of epidemic meningococcal meningitis in sub-Saharan Africa may be amenable to more traditional vaccine approaches, using meningococcal polysaccharides conjugated to protein carriers. The issues here are not the vaccines per se, but their cost, the logistics and politics of their deployment, and the organizational infrastructure needed to bring them to the groups who need them the most in these developing parts of the world.

Group B meningococci continue to pose problems for vaccinologists. As we have seen, despite the fact that the core of these organisms is surrounded by a capsular polysaccharide—as is the case with other meningococcal serogroups—their polysaccharide coat does not engender protective antibody responses when formulated into a vaccine. Instead, the human immune system turns its attention elsewhere—"tolerates" it—because it looks too much like parts of its "self," and the immune system is genetically programmed not to attack its own cells and tissues. With a polysaccharide type of vaccine out of contention, researchers have looked for other targets within the bacterium against which to direct immune responses.

The outer membrane of the group B meningococcus—the layer that separates the interior of the bacterium from the outside world—contains a number of different molecules that assist the germ in its efforts to evade the human immune system. Infectious diseases frequently result from such a chess game; a microbe struggles to survive in the hostile environment of its host, and in order to do this, it generally employs multiple strategies to avoid getting caught up in the body's defenses. The group B meningococcus is no stranger to intrigue.

Studding the outer membrane of group B meningococcus are various proteins that serve an array of the germ's priorities—evasion of the immune system highest among these. During invasion into the bloodstream, the bacterium releases microscopic 'packets' containing portions of these outer membrane proteins in an attempt to divert the host's immune responses.[4] As a countermove, various experimental vaccines over the past two decades have used the protein contents of these packages to provoke an antibody response that targets group B meningococci. These vaccine strategies have resulted in only moderate success, in large part because the outer membrane proteins of various strains of these bacteria are moving targets—they are highly diverse and frequently change their appearance—rendering it difficult to predict the effective components of any one single vaccine.

Another, innovative approach to identifying components of the group B meningococcus that could potentially serve as effective targets of a protective immune response has taken the opposite tack to that of traditional vaccine development—a "molecular" one. Historically, the search for a vaccine has begun by growing a germ in culture, breaking it down chemically into its specific components, and deciphering immune responses to these pieces—usually by injecting the various parts into animals and testing them for their ability to provoke an immune response that is protective against infection. Sometimes, as with pathogens that solely infect humans, immune responses can only be understood by testing human serum for its ability to kill bacteria, since it is not necessarily feasible or advisable to inject the pieces into people.

Once an immune response is identified as being protective against a certain pathogen—such as antibody targeting the polysaccharide capsule of group C meningococci—vaccinologists seek to find or create a mechanism to induce those same protective immune responses in humans. That is precisely the strategy employed by the WRAIR group in the late 1960s that resulted in the first effective meningococcal vaccines. But a decade ago Rino Rappuoli, the global head of vaccine research for the large pharmaceutical company Novartis, turned this strategy on its ear and created a new one—"reverse vaccinology"—that looks at vaccine protection from an entirely different perspective.

Rappuoli deduced that to develop a vaccine with broad activity against group B meningococci and all of its various strains—a "universal" vaccine—highly conserved protein molecules of the bacteria would have to be identified. Why proteins? Because it seemed clear from all that was known about group B, that the polysaccharide capsule was not an option. Once the actual DNA sequence—the "genome"—of group B meningococcus was known, the precise order of the genes that encode for specific proteins of the bacteria was available for study. This allowed Rappuoli's group to explore the coded proteins—like miners looking for rare gems—using computer-based algorithms to pick out the ones that met their criteria as possible targets of the immune system—ones that would have the best potential chance to generate antibody responses.[5] Through this rapid "genome mining," they identified five proteins on the outer surface of the group B meningococcus that fit their criteria, combined them into a vaccine formulation, and successfully induced high levels of protective antibodies against the bacteria by injecting this vaccine into mice.

The "holy grail" of vaccinology is to develop vaccines that are effective against every possible strain or variation of a specific pathogen or group of pathogens. To do this would likely require a vaccine containing "universal"—conserved—elements derived from the surface of a germ that induces an effective immune response. For groups A and C meningococci, this was first made possible—40 years ago—by creating vaccines that directed the immune response against the conserved, polysaccharide capsule that surrounds these bacteria. For group B meningococci, vaccines containing a cocktail of various proteins identified by mining the bacteria's genome—with or without the addition of little packets containing outer membrane proteins—have been tested in children and adults and found to be safe and able to induce protective antibody against multiple strains of group B. Such vaccines have also shown early promise in infants—the group at the greatest risk of meningococcal disease.[6] The "holy grail" may be visible in the distance.

Unlike the pure laboratory approach that has characterized an as-yet incomplete search for effective vaccines against group B meningococci, the solution to the enormous, recurring problem of epidemic meningococcal meningitis—generally group A disease—in the countries of the African "meningitis belt" appears to be clearly delineated, although difficult to deliver. This is more of a traditional, brute force type of vaccine dilemma: how to formulate a relatively low-cost, highly effective, safe vaccine that can be deployed to all children and young adults—basically the majority of the population—across the vast reaches of both densely populated cities and sparsely inhabited villages in some of the poorest and most politically unstable places on earth.

The area first described by the famous French epidemiologist Lapeyssonnie in 1963—the "meningitis belt"—extends across the northern, sub-Saharan part of the continent from Senegal to Ethiopia, and it comprises all or part of fifteen countries. It is home to more than 300 million people—the population of the entire U.S. In the 1990s, hundreds of thousands of cases of meningococcal meningitis occurred there—200,000 in 1996 alone—prompting the World Health Organization (WHO) to convene an expert panel to strategize about the potential for large-scale vaccination efforts there to stave off the massive burden of deaths, childhood hearing loss, seizures, cognitive deficits, social disruption, and economic catastrophe that generally attended the outbreaks and would invariably accompany the next epidemic wave. What eventually emerged in 2001 from this planning process—with the endorsement of international experts and African public health officials—was a Gates Foundation-funded partnership between the WHO and a three-decade-old nonprofit organization based in Seattle.

Initially launched with a reproductive health focus, the Program for Appropriate Technology in Health—now just PATH—had evolved from these humble roots to its ambitious focus on improving overall global health. Their mission—involving work in 70 countries—is based on an entrepreneurial and technology-based approach to the design and deployment of "high-impact, low-cost solutions" to important issues ranging from vaccines against epidemic diseases to bed net distribution to prevent malaria.[7] Their methods are heavily steeped in collaborative programs involving businesses and international communities in order to actually bring the solutions directly to the people on the ground who need them.

To solve the daunting, 150-year-old problem of epidemic meningococcal disease in sub-Saharan Africa, the newly minted WHO–PATH collaboration with the African countries of the "meningitis belt" would have to work under complex epidemiologic, scientific, economic, and political conditions that often veered into ambiguity—a situation both parties were accustomed to through years of field work in developing countries. But first, their initiative would require a leader not only experienced in infectious diseases and public health issues but also one who was highly skilled in nurturing relationships and had the practical sense and personal drive to accomplish this mission under difficult circumstances. They turned to Dr. Marc LaForce, a 35-year veteran of public health with a penchant for dealing with the types of thorny problems with which he would soon be faced.

LaForce's career trajectory had covered a lot of ground in classic infectious diseases laboratory research, clinical medicine, epidemiology, and international public health since his medical residency on the Harvard Service at Boston City Hospital in the mid-1960s. Following a two-year stint as an Epidemic Intelligence Service Officer working on meningitis surveillance with the forerunner of the Centers for Disease Control in Atlanta, he returned to Boston City Hospital as a research fellow in infectious diseases at the Channing and Thorndike Laboratories. Then came leadership positions in academic medicine, interspersed with a variety of consultancies and tours with various international public health agencies. He worked on the smallpox eradication program in Bangladesh in 1975; WHO polio surveillance and the efforts for universal childhood immunization in Asia and Africa in the 1970s and 1980s; and for two decades with the U.S. Agency for International Development (USAID), WHO, and the United Nations Children's Fund (UNICEF)—in Africa, India, and around the world—developing partnerships and building relationships to enhance childhood immunization against polio, tetanus, and a host of other routinely preventable diseases.

He had been hearing about the possible development of a major initiative towards an international, meningitis vaccine effort in sub-Saharan Africa while directing USAID's child survival project in early 2001. A few months later—just one month after being offered the job—he was again on the ground in Africa, as the Director of the Meningitis Vaccine Project (MVP).[8] The project's overarching goal was not a modest one: the elimination of epidemic meningococcal meningitis—by definition, group A disease—from sub-Saharan Africa; their time frame to reach that goal, also ambitious—fifteen years.

The vision was clear; however, the path to it required much more than purchasing existing vaccines and organizing a deployment strategy. This, alone, would be highly complex given the constellation of conditions that exist in the region. But this project involved a massive undertaking in an economic market outside of the usual business opportunities that interest vaccine manufacturers, making the acquisition of a suitable vaccine problem number one.

LaForce and his team spent the better part of the first year with the MVP on the ground trying to understand the problem from the African perspective. Working with his WHO counterpart, they made several trips to Francophone countries of West Africa. LaForce—a fluent French speaker—was repeatedly told, "don't develop a product we cannot afford." In order to sustain a meningococcal vaccination effort in "belt" countries, the vaccine would need to cost less than 50 cents per dose—several orders of magnitude less than the cost of commercially available conjugate vaccines.

LaForce believes that the key turning point in the MVP strategy was the decision to develop a "homegrown" meningococcal conjugate vaccine. This leap of faith — taken in the fall of 2002 — ran counter to the easier, usual approach of setting up a contract with a major pharmaceutical company that was already working in the conjugate vaccine business. 'Big Pharma' had decided not to pursue this market for economic reasons; the MVP would need to acquire their meningococcal vaccine the hard way.

The MVP team broke down the development of a new African meningococcal conjugate vaccine into three essential, interrelated steps. First, they needed to obtain the raw materials for a polysaccharide–protein conjugate product — large quantities of vaccine-grade, meningococcal group A polysaccharide and large quantities of a carrier protein. Tetanus toxoid was chosen as the carrier protein because it would be an independently useful component of any vaccine in this population — who were at risk for tetanus as well. Then, they would have to find a company willing to accept the transfer of technology derived from the two pieces created from step one in order to produce a conjugate vaccine. Finally, the MVP team would have to resolve the "intellectual property" issue as to who would actually own this new conjugation recipe, as existing pharmaceutical companies that made conjugate vaccines were not anxious to share their proprietary technology.

For the raw materials for the project, an established manufacturer in Amsterdam agreed to produce the group A polysaccharide. Tetanus toxoid came from the Serum Institute of India, Ltd., an experienced vaccine producer boasting a four decade-long track record in the business of making protein antitoxins and antivenoms for snakebites. The third piece came from scientists at the U.S. Food and Drug Administration who had developed an innovative conjugation method. A technology transfer agreement stipulated that PATH would own the technology but sublicense it to the Serum Institute of India in what amounted to a "win–win".[8] Through the many administrative steps, it became increasingly clear that this was both a project people cared about and an important business opportunity for the Indian-owned company looking to break into the conjugate vaccine market. The Serum Institute of India, Ltd. would manufacture the vaccine — MenAfriVac™ — to be used in Africa.[9]

Through a series of mandated but scientifically necessary studies, the vaccine's safety was assured and its ability to generate strong antibody responses directed against the polysaccharide capsule in African children — as young as one year of age — and young adults was demonstrated. Additionally, it was hoped that the vaccine would generate herd immunity — preventing the bacteria from being carried in the noses and throats of people — thus providing hope that vaccinating one to 29-year-olds might also protect unvaccinated infants and adults over 30 years old by reducing their exposure to the bacteria. In late 2009, the vaccine received market authorization from the Drug Controller of India; six months later, MenAfriVac™ was "prequalified" by WHO — meaning that it could be purchased by UNICEF for distribution in the "meningitis belt." Plans were developed to deploy it in the first, comprehensive meningococcal vaccination of an African "belt" country.[10]

Burkina Faso, known as Upper Volta at the time Lapeyssonnie wrote his now famous monograph describing the African "meningitis belt" 50 years ago, lies at the heart of the area of highest meningococcal disease risk. In a country of more than 15 million people, most are under the age of 30. An epidemic of group A meningitis five years previously had caused more than 45,000 cases of the disease there. Burkina Faso, Mali—its neighbor to the northwest, and Niger—to its immediate east were selected by the MVP to be early adopters of the new vaccine on the basis of their risk for epidemic disease, the presence of robust meningitis surveillance systems, and supportive health ministries. However, only the Burkinabes were committed to vaccinating their one to 29-year-olds—nearly three-quarters of the country's entire population—before the end of calendar year 2010. Hence, this country was the first in which MenAfriVac™ was deployed.

In a ten-day period in early December 2010, the national campaign safely vaccinated more than 11.4 million children and young adults—one hundred percent of the targeted populations—in Burkina Faso.[8] These staggering statistics speak to the extraordinary immunization infrastructure that was in place there. Such a high level of vaccine acceptance by the population suggested the interplay of multiple, contributing factors: high levels of concern about the disease among the public led to a desire to receive "the good vaccine"; a well-organized, well-informed communication plan, initiated two years before vaccine introduction; and strong political support on the ground, exemplified by the country's President presiding over the campaign's launch.[8]

The massive, countrywide, meningococcal vaccination effort in Burkina Faso in late 2010 had a high probability of success from the start based on the expertise and experience of the MVP partnership. PATH took the lead in vaccine development, which required creative alliances, technology-based entrepreneurship, and political maneuvering. WHO was responsible for disease surveillance systems and vaccine deployment, areas in which they could boast a long and successful track record—from smallpox eradication to measles and beyond.

As of April 2012, nearly 55 million children and young adults in at least six "meningitis belt" countries—Burkina Faso, Chad, Cameroon, Mali, Niger, and Nigeria—have received MenAfriVac™. The MVP plans call for vaccinating an additional 265 million people across sub-Saharan Africa by 2016.[11] Although it is too early to evaluate the true effectiveness of the vaccine in preventing epidemic meningococcal meningitis in the region, early reports suggest that despite ongoing outbreaks in non-vaccinated areas, the vaccine appears to have—at least during the first year—stopped the disease in its tracks.

The ultimate hope in Africa would be to develop and deploy—in a similar fashion as has been done with group A meningococcal vaccine—a conjugate meningococcal vaccine that covers the other main, epidemic serogroups of concern there. Based on the efforts already underway, this would appear to be an achievable goal. Perhaps the most important result from the first decade of the MVP in sub-Saharan Africa is that it has opened up a new way to develop and deploy very low-cost products without having to rely on 'Big Pharma' and by doing so empowers future large-scale public health interventions throughout the world.

The 200-year-old history of epidemic meningococcal meningitis parallels the history of modern medicine and the development of public health. Its early history in the pivotal nineteenth century occurred in the context of the establishment of the germ theory of disease causation, the rise of microbiology and immunology as distinct disciplines of science, and the inception of vaccines against diverse pathogens. The second century of meningococcal disease—which has only recently ended—witnessed the evolution of specific treatments for infectious diseases. First came serum therapy, applied to such diseases as diphtheria, tetanus, meningococcal meningitis, and subsequently pneumococcal pneumonia. Then, in the late 1930s, antibacterial chemotherapy—sulfa drugs, penicillin, and a slew of others that followed—entered the picture and dramatically changed the landscape. For a brief historical moment, it seemed as though infectious diseases would be relegated to the dustbin of history. But that, of course, was wishful thinking; microbes are formidable foes.

Once it became clear that the only definitive solution to infectious diseases was to prevent their occurrence in the first place, the development of vaccines gained adherents as the best approach to achieve this goal. For meningococcal meningitis, the history of vaccines officially dates to the revelations of the WRAIR group in the late 1960s and their creation of the first, effective polysaccharide vaccine for this disease. Over the ensuing four decades, incremental and at times, major advances in these vaccines were accomplished. The advent of conjugate vaccines held the promise of improved effectiveness in the very youngest and most vulnerable of potential meningococcal victims—infants.

Although there remain significant needs to fill with regard to the worldwide prevention of epidemic meningococcal meningitis, we appear to be closing in on that ultimate objective. The MVP has shown that it may be possible to end the two-century-old recurring nightmare of epidemic disease in Africa through innovative vaccine approaches. Group B disease, which has eluded a vaccine solution because of its ability to deceive the human immune system, may be in our vaccine sights. Paul Offit, the Chief of Infectious Diseases at the Children's Hospital of Philadelphia and a leading proponent of vaccines, believes that "by 2017 we should have—with the technologies currently underway—a viable and effective group B vaccine, and with a strategy of routine immunizations, we may be able to eliminate meningococci as a significant cause of human disease".[12] As we enter the early years of the third century of epidemic meningococcal meningitis, there is the real possibility that they could represent the final act for this worldwide plague. And that would be a great benefit to all of us.

Epilogue

The saga of epidemic meningococcal meningitis, traced through its more than two centuries of documented history, illuminates many facets of medical science. Although probably not a disease of antiquity—like smallpox, measles, or anthrax—meningococcal disease has much to teach us about the scientific process, medical research, and human suffering. It is perhaps an especially instructive infectious disease as its history parallels that of the rise of modern medicine. In its social context, the story of meningococcal meningitis covers familiar—but critically important—ground as both an active participant and a witness to epochal events of the last 200 years.

What does the history of meningococcal meningitis teach us about medical research in general? First, that medical science is a multinational process. Pasteur and Koch were both informed by centuries of their inquisitive predecessors from all parts of the world. The findings that emanated from their laboratories in Paris and Berlin, respectively, led—among many other discoveries—to the advent of microbiology and immunology as distinct fields and, subsequently, to the identification of the bacterial cause of epidemic meningitis. The research models they presided over in Europe greatly influenced the inception of America's Rockefeller Institute, leading directly to the systematic application of the first effective treatment—serum therapy—for meningococcal meningitis.

Disease, like science, is also multinational. In the case of epidemic meningococcal meningitis, the greatest burden of disease occurs in Africa, but periodic outbreaks and sporadic episodes of the infection occur throughout the world. Although different in volume and scope, human anguish—death and permanent disability—engendered by meningococcal disease is also a worldwide phenomenon.

The story of meningococcal meningitis teaches that medical science is multidisciplinary. Major breakthroughs in medical research—"game changers"—are enabled by the accrual of incremental advances across multiple other fields. As we have seen, the discovery of antibacterial drugs, such as sulfa, only became possible after 80 years of progress in industrial dyes, synthetic organic chemistry, microbiology, and pharmaceutical research. In order to decipher the identity of the "specific soluble substance," Avery, a physician scientist, had to find a crackerjack organic chemist—Heidelberger—with whom to collaborate. Their combined, extraordinary talents caused a paradigm shift that left an indelible mark on biology and lighted the way for polysaccharide vaccines. Thus, the invention of the first, effective meningococcal vaccine by the WRAIR group in the late 1960s did not occur in a vacuum; it was intricately linked to a half-century of basic and applied research.

The 200-year recorded history of epidemic meningitis instructs us that medical science is multigenerational. It is generally slow, pain-staking work with many more setbacks than successes. And in the broader context of human disease, the journey to at least partially effective meningococcal vaccines—for most serogroups—has been relatively brisk. Smallpox terrorized humans for thousands of years before it was finally brought under complete control—eradicated—as a cause of natural disease.

A major factor in the multigenerational aspect of medical and scientific advances is that progress is directly correlated with technical advances in the laboratory—and these take time. The very existence of microscopic germs, suspected as early as the sixteenth century, could not be demonstrated until van Leeuwenhoek's work with his primitive microscopes a century later. It would take another 200 years—until Koch developed ways to grow bacteria in culture—before a causal relationship between germs and human disease could be proven. With meningococcal meningitis, newer generation, conjugate vaccine technologies—40 years after the invention of the first polysaccharide meningococcal vaccine—have improved the outlook for disease prevention in children. However, effective vaccine solutions for the most vulnerable ones—infants—and the most deceptive meningococcal type—group B—remain elusive.

Finally, the story of meningococcal meningitis illustrates the humbling nature of medical science. The early success of the massive Meningitis Vaccine Project in sub-Saharan Africa holds the promise of a future without meningitis for millions of young Africans. There, cost, logistics, and leadership remain the greatest challenges. Nonetheless, despite the best efforts of modern medicine and the availability of an effective vaccine, Michael Gomes, a healthy, active teenager living in Massachusetts, rapidly succumbed to the disease in a state-of-the-art, hospital intensive care unit. Such tragedies still occur and remind us that while we may be close to the final act of meningococcal meningitis, we are not yet ready to claim final victory.

Source Notes

Instead of using footnotes in the text, I have chosen to list all citations here, as is the standard in scientific medical writing. The citations contain a combination of published scientific papers, articles from the lay press, book sources, and interviews conducted by the author. For each chapter, I have annotated some of the most useful of these sources for those interested in further reading on the subjects. After, I provide a selected bibliography of important sources; many of these are referred to in the text, while others provided important background information for the subject matter and were used for this purpose only.

Chapter 1: Origins

Probably the best "big picture" perspective on the evolution and development of human societies is found in Diamond (1997). Some of his other works, not cited here, delve even deeper into this theme. Hopkins (1983) and Cantor (2002) provide insightful and extensive commentaries on the far-reaching impact of two of the most historically important diseases—smallpox and plague, respectively. Hopkins (1983) is a must-read for anyone interested in the history of that scourge of antiquity—smallpox.

1. Diamond J. Guns, germs, and steel: the fates of human societies. New York: W.W. Norton & Company; 1997.
2. Conrad LI, Neve M, Nutton V, et al. The Western medical tradition 800 BC to AD 1800. Cambridge: Cambridge University Press; 1995.
3. Kalish ML, Robbins KE, Pieniazek D, et al. Recombinant viruses and early global HIV-1 epidemic. Emerg Infect Dis. 2004;10:1227–34.
4. Stevens J, Blixt O, Tumpey TM, et al. Structure and receptor specificity of the hemagglutinin from an H5N1 influenza. Virus. 2006;312:404–10.
5. Herzog C, Salès N, Etchegaray N, et al. Tissue distribution of bovine spongiform encephalopathy agent in primates after intravenous or oral infection. Lancet. 2004;363:422–7.
6. Margaret H, Ng L, Lau KM, et al. Association of human-leukocyte antigen class 1 (B*0703) and class 2 (DRB1*0301) genotypes with susceptibility and resistance to the development of severe acute respiratory syndrome. J Infect Dis. 2004;190:515–8.
7. Sherman IW. Twelve diseases that changed our world. Washington DC: ASM Press; 2007.

8. Brier B. Infectious disease in ancient Egypt. Infect Dis Clin North Am. 2004;18:17–27.

9. Cunha BA. The cause of the plague of Athens: plague, typhoid, typhus, smallpox, or measles? Infect Dis Clin North Am. 2004;18:29–43.

10. Fears JR. The plague under Marcus Aurelius and the decline and fall of the Roman Empire. Infect Dis Clin North Am. 2004;18:65–77.

11. Zinsser H. Rats, lice and history. Boston: Little, Brown and Company; 1934.

12. Trevisanato SI. Did an epidemic of tularemia in Ancient Egypt affect the course of world history? Med Hypotheses. 2004;63:905–10.

13. Asad S, Artenstein AW. Occupational plague. In: Wright WE, editor. Couturier's occupational and environmental infectious diseases. 2nd ed. Beverly Farms, MA: OEM Press; 2009.

14. Drancourt M, Raoult D. Molecular insights into the history of plague. Microbes Infect. 2002;4:105–9.

15. Cantor NF. In the wake of the plague: the black death and the world it made. New York: Perennial; 2002.

16. Galvani AP, Slatkin M. Evaluating plague and smallpox as historical selective pressures for the CCR5-Delta 32 HIV-resistance allele. Proc Natl Acad Sci USA. 2003;100:15276–9.

17. McNeill WH. Plagues and people. New York: Doubleday; 1976.

18. Cook ND. Born to die: disease and New World conquest, 1492–1650. Cambridge: Cambridge University Press; 1998.

19. Hopkins DR. The greatest killer: smallpox in history. Chicago: University of Chicago Press; 1983.

20. Artenstein AW, Opal JM, Opal SM, et al. History of U.S. Military contributions to the study of vaccines against infectious diseases. Mil Med. 2005;170:3–11.

21. Murphy J. An American plague: the true and terrifying story of the yellow fever epidemic of 1793. New York: Clarion Books; 2003.

22. McCullough D. The path between the seas: the creation of the Panama Canal 1870–1914. New York: Simon and Shuster; 1977.

23. Panum PL. Observations made during the epidemic of measles on the Faroe Islands in the year 1846 [English edition: Panum PL (1940) (Delta Omega Society, trans)]. New York: American Public Health Association; 1847.

Chapter 2: The Art and Science of Germs

The relatively brief, sixty-year history of microbiology—as it was in the 1930s—is beautifully articulated in the work of Bulloch (1936). Specific biographies of seminal scientists and the contributions they made to the development of a science of microbes are best recounted in Dobell (1960), Nuland (1979), Johnson (2002), Money (2007), Debré (1994), and Brock (1988). The work of Bynum (1994) describes the status and development of medicine and science in the pivotal nineteenth century; perhaps Johnson (2002) paints the most memorable and vivid picture of disease pestilence in that newly industrialized society.

1. Bulloch W. The history of bacteriology: University of London Heath Clark Lectures, 1936. New York, NY: Dover Publications, Inc., 1938.

2. Leviticus. In Plaut WG, ed. The Torah: A modern commentary. Union of American Hebrew Congregations; New York, 1981;11:1–23.

3. Fracastorius H. De sympathia et antipathia rerum, liber unus, De contagione et contagiosis morbis et curatione, lib. Iii, Venetiis, 1546 [Wilmer Cave Wright, English trans]. New York: G.P. Putnam's sons; 1930.

4. Quétel C. The history of syphilis. Johns Hopkins University Press; Baltimore, 1990.

5. Dobell C. Antony van Leeuwenhoek and his "Little Animals": being some account of the Father of Protozoology and Bacteriology and his multifarious discoveries in these disciplines. New York: Dover Publications Inc.; 1960.

6. Corliss JO. A salute to Antony van Leeuwenhoek of Delft, most versatile 17th century founding father of protistology. Protist. 2002;153:177–90.

7. Gensini GF, Conti AA. The evolution of the concept of "fever" in the history of medicine: from pathological picture per se to clinical epiphenomenon (and vice versa). J Infect. 2004;49:85–7.

8. Wyklicky H, Skopec M. Ignaz Philipp Semmelweis, the prophet of bacteriology. Infect Control. 1983;4:367–70.

9. Nuland SB. Germs, childbed fever, and the strange story of Ignac Semmelweis. New York: W. W. Norton and Co.; 2003.

10. Nuland SB. The enigma of Semmelweis-an interpretation. J Hist Med Allied Sci. 1979; 34:255–72

11. Carpenter CCJ. The Jeremiah Metzger lecture. Myths, mandarins and molecules: the cautionary tale of cholera. Trans Am Clin Climatol Assoc. 1981;92:167–93.

12. Snow J. On the mode of communication of cholera. Churchill; London, 1855.

13. Johnson S. The ghost map: the story of London's most terrifying epidemic and how it changed science, cities and the modern world. New York: Riverhead; 2002.

14. Sherman IW. Twelve diseases that changed our world. Washington DC: ASM Press, 2007.

15. Money NP. The triumph of the fungi: a rotten history. New York: Oxford University Press; 2007.

16. Berkeley MJ. Observations, botanical and physiological, on the potato murrain. J Horticult Soc Lond. 1846;1:9–34.

17. Gest H. Fresh views of the 17th century discoveries by Hooke and van Leeuwenhoek. Microbe. 2007;2:483–8.

18. Redi of Aresso, Francesco. Experiments on the generation of insects [Mab Bigelow, trans]. Chicago: The Open Court Publishing Company; 1909.

19. Debré P. Louis Pasteur [English edition: Debré P (1998) Louis Pasteur (Forster E, trans)]. Baltimore: The Johns Hopkins University Press; 994.

20. Lister J. On a new method of treating compound fracture, abscess, and so forth; with observations on the conditions of suppuration. In: Brock TD, editor. Milestones in microbiology: 1546 to 1940 [T.D. Brock, trans]. Washington DC: ASM Press; 1999. p. 83–5.

21. Bynum WF. Science and the practice of medicine in the nineteenth century. New York: Cambridge University Press; 1994.

22. Harding-Rains AJ. Joseph Lister and antisepsis. Sussex, UK: Priory Press; 1977.

23. Wangesteen ON, Wangesteen SD. The rise of surgery, from a empiric craft to scientific discipline. Minneapolis: University of Minnesota Press; 1978.

24. Brock TD. Robert Koch: a life in medicine and bacteriology. Washington DC: American Society for Microbiology; 1988.

25. Petri, RJ. A Minor Modification of the plating technique of Koch. In: Brock TD, editor. Milestones in microbiology: 1546 to 1940 [T.D. Brock, trans]. Washington DC: ASM Press; 1999. p. 218–9.

26. Ryan F. The forgotten plague: how the battle against tuberculosis was won — and lost. Little, Brown and Company; United Kingdom, 1992.

27. Dubos R, Dubos J. The white plague. Boston: Little Brown; 1956.

28. Kaufmann SH, Winau F. From bacteriology to immunology: the dualism of specificity. Nat Immunol. 2005;6:1063–6.

Chapter 3: A Singular Disease

Sydenham's work (1788) is the definitive compendium of clinical medicine—as it was appreciated in the seventeenth century. The monograph by North (1811) provides a complete collection of many of the earliest American experiences with meningococcal disease and provides some of the most clear and detailed descriptions of its clinical manifestations. The truly "local" flavor—the cases occurred in Connecticut, and the "remarks" that are appended are derived from various physicians and medical society meetings in southern New England in the first decade of the nineteenth century—permeates this impressive collection. Similarly, the monograph by Councilman (1898) contains a virtual treasure trove of historical, epidemiological, clinical, and pathological information on the disease, as it was understood at the end of its first century.

1. Sydenham T. The works of Thomas Sydenham, M.D. on Acute and chronic diseases: wherein their histories and modes of cure, as recited by him, are delivered with accuracy and perspicuity. To which are Subjoined notes, corrective and explanatory, from the most eminent. London: G.G.H. and J. Robinson, W. Otridge, S. Hayes, and E. Newbery; 1788.
2. Brock TD. Robert Koch: a life in medicine and bacteriology. Washington DC: American Society for Microbiology; 1988.
3. Opal SM. A brief history of microbiology and immunology. In: Artenstein AW, editor. Vaccines: a biography. New York: Springer; 2010. p. 31–56.
4. Rivers TM. Filterable viruses. J Bacteriol. 1927;14:217–58.
5. Weichselbaum A. Ueber die Aetiologie der akuten Menigitis cerebro-spinalis. Fortschr Med. 1887;5:573–83.
6. Vieusseux G. Mémoire sur la maladie qui a regné à Genève au printemps de 1805. J Med Chi Pharmacol. 1805;11:163–93.
7. Danielson L, Mann E. The history of a singular and very mortal disease, which lately made its appearance in Medfield. Med Agric Reg. 1806;1:65–9.
8. Vaughan VC. Cerebrospinal meningitis. In: Epidemiology and public health. St. Louis: C.V. Mosby Co.; 1922. p. 528–98.
9. Murchison C. On the cerebro-spinal symptoms and lesions of typhus fever, and on the relation of typhus to epidemic cerebro-spinal meningitis. The Lancet. 1865;1:417–8.
10. Anonymous. Cerebro-spinal meningitis. Br Med J. 1865;1:8–12.
11. Grady FJ. Some early American reports on meningitis. J His Med Allied Sci. 1965;20:27–32.
12. North E. A treatise on a malignant epidemic commonly called spotted fever. New York: T. & J. Swords; 1811.
13. Steiner, PE. Disease in the civil war: natural biological warfare in 1861–1865. Springfield, IL: Charles C. Thomas Publisher; 1968.
14. Councilman WT, Mallory FB, Wright JH. Epidemic cerebro-spinal meningitis and its relation to other forms of meningitis. Boston, MA: Report of the State Board of Health of MA; 1898. p.1–178.
15. Ligon BL. Albert Ludwig Sigesmund Neisser: discoverer of the cause of gonorrhea. Semin Pediatr Infect Dis. 2005;16:336–41.
16. Feldman HA. Meningococcus and gonococcus: never the twain…well, hardly ever. N Engl J Med. 1971;285:518–20.

Chapter 4: A Very Mortal Disease

Both Thigpen (2011) and Stephens (2007) provide excellent, recent reviews of the epidemiology and pathophysiology of meningococcal disease. Lapeyssonnie's famous monograph (1963) establishes the epidemiology of meningitis in Africa—the "meningitis belt"—for the first time; the important history of the disease on that continent is reviewed in detail by Greenwood (2006). The book by Tracey (2006) represents a detailed, yet easily understandable account of the battle that is waged within the human body between infecting organisms and the immune system. Written for a lay readership, he uses the case—one of his own as a newly minted surgical resident—of a young child victim of a severe burn and the subsequent hospital events, including overwhelming infections, that befell her.

1. Peters, FE. The Hajj: the Muslim pilgrimage to Mecca and the holy places. Princeton, NJ: Princeton University Press; 1994.
2. Khan MA. Outbreaks of meningococcal meningitis during Hajj: changing face of an old enemy. J Pak Med Assoc. 2003;53:3–7.
3. Thigpen MC, Whitney CG, Messonnier NE, et al. Bacterial meningitis in the United States, 1998–2007. N Engl J Med. 2011;364:2016–25.
4. Lapeyssonnie L. La méningite cérébro-spinale en Afrique. Bull World Health Organ. 1963;28:Suppl:1–114.
5. Greenwood B. 100 years of epidemic meningitis in West Africa—has anything changed? Trop Med Int Health. 2006;11:773–80.
6. McGahey K. Report on an outbreak of epidemic cerebrospinal meningitis in Zungeru during February and March 1905. J Trop Med. 1905;8:210–6.
7. Greenwood B. Meningococcal meningitis in Africa. Trans R Soc Trop Med Hyg. 1999;93:341–53.
8. Stephens DS, Greenwood B, Brandtzaeg. Epidemic meningitis, meningococcaemia, and *Neisseria meningitidis*. Lancet. 2007;369:2196–210.
9. Goldschneider I, Gotschlich EC, Artenstein MS. Human immunity to the meningococcus. I. The role of humoral antibodies. J Exp Med. 1969;129:1307–26.
10. Tracey KJ. Fatal sequence: the killer within. New York: Dana Press; 2006.
11. Osler W. The Cavendish Lecture on the etiology and diagnosis of cerebro-spinal fever. Br Med J. 1899;1:1517–28.
12. Rosenstein NE, Perkins BA, Stephens DS, Popovic T, Hughes JM. Meningococcal disease. N Engl J Med. 2001;344:1378–88.
13. North E. A treatise on a malignant epidemic commonly called spotted fever. New York: T. & J. Swords; 1811.

Chapter 5: Early Approaches at Therapy

Chernow's Titan (1998) provides a compelling, highly readable, information-packed biography of the complex, multi-faceted Rockefeller Sr. The books of both Brown (1979) and Corner (1964) describe the key players—including Gates—in the development of the concept and implementation of the Rockefeller Institute vision. Corner's work is clearly a 'company' version of events, but it usefully fills in the necessary names and dates. Bliss (1999) is the definitive work on perhaps the greatest

physician—Osler—in modern medical history. Details on the life and times of Simon
Flexner are recounted in many of the above sources but also in the book by his son—
the author J.T. Flexner (1993) that examines, in parallel fashion, the divergent paths
of his famous mother and father. The scientific reports of Simon Flexner (1906, 1907,
1908, 1913) are important reading as they demonstrate the path of antimeningococcal antiserum from bench to bedside and also provide a sense of just how impressive
the survival benefit was to patients suffering from an otherwise lethal disease who
prior to this therapeutic intervention had little hope.

1. Brown RE. Rockefeller medicine men: medicine and capitalism in America. Berkeley, CA:
   University of California Press; 1979.
2. Chernow RE. Titan: the life of John D. Rockefeller, Sr. New York: Random House Inc.;
   1998.
3. Bliss M. William Osler: a life in medicine. New York: Oxford University Press; 1999.
4. Flexner S, Flexner JT. William Henry Welch and the heroic age of American medicine.
   New York: Viking Press; 1941.
5. Corner GW. A history of the Rockefeller Institute 1901–1953. New York: The Rockefeller
   Institute Press; 1964.
6. Rous P. Simon Flexner and medical discovery. Science. 1948;107:611–3.
7. Flexner JT. An American saga: the story of Helen Thomas and Simon Flexner. New York:
   Fordham University Press; 1993.
8. Darlington T. Cerebro-spinal meningitis. Trans Am Climatol Assoc. 1906;22:56–70.
9. Flexner S. Contributions to the biology of *Diplococcus intracellularis*. J Exp Med.
   1907;9:105–41.
10. Frederiks JAM, Koehler PJ. The first lumbar puncture. J Hist Neurosci. 1997;6:147–53.
11. Pearce JMS. Walter Essex Wynter, Quincke, and lumbar puncture. J Neurol Neurosurg
    Psychiatry. 1994;57:179.
12. Flexner S. Concerning a serum-therapy for experimental infection with *Diplococcus intracel-
    lularis*. J Exp Med. 1907;9:168–85.
13. Grabenstein JD. Toxoid vaccines. In: Artenstein AW, editor. Vaccines: a biography. New York:
    Springer; 2010.
14. Oliver WW. The man who lived for tomorrow. New York: E.P. Dutton and Co., Inc.; 1941.
15. Flexner S. Experimental cerebro-spinal meningitis in monkeys. J Exp Med. 1907;9:142–67.
16. Flexner S. Experimental cerebrospinal meningitis and its serum treatment. JAMA.
    1906;47:560–6.
17. Jochmann G. Versuche zur Serodiagnostik und Serotherapie der epidemischen Genickstarre.
    Deutsche Medizinische Wochenschrift. 1906;32:788–93.
18. Flexner S, Jobling JW. Serum treatment of epidemic cerebro-spinal meningitis. J Exp Med.
    1908;10:141–203.
19. Flexner S, Jobling JW. An analysis of four hundred cases of epidemic meningitis treated with
    the anti-meningitis serum. J Exp Med. 1908;10:690–733.
20. Flexner S. The results of the serum treatment in thirteen hundred cases of epidemic meningitis.
    J Exp Med. 1913;15:553–75.
21. Sophian A. Epidemic cerebrospinal meningitis. St Louis: CV Mosby Co.; 1913.
22. Finland M. The serum treatment of lobar pneumonia. N Engl J Med. 1930;202:1244–7.

Chapter 6: Antibiotics and Survival of the Fittest

The most thorough scientific histories of the origins and development of the sulfa class of antimicrobials are the work of Lesch (1981, 2007); Travis (1993) and Garfield (2001) provide important background information on the history of the dye industry, essential for understanding the relationships of coal tar, synthetic dyes, and pharmaceuticals. The history of Bayer is a fascinating one—although beyond the scope of this work—and one that is fraught with source bias. The Bayer Website provides an interesting and not unexpected perspective on their own history, of course minimizing patent controversies and the "troubles" during the Nazi era. Nowhere to be found there is mention of its marketing of heroin as a cough remedy. The story behind I. G. Farben and their complex, complicit relationship with Hitler's regime is well documented in Jeffreys (2008) and more dramatically retold in Borkin (1978). Parascandola (1981) does an excellent job of explaining the scientific basis of "chemotherapy" and Ehrlich's vision as conceived in the early years of the twentieth century. Perhaps the best source—and most colorfully written—through which to place the sulfa drugs in their historical context is Galdston (1943). Finally, for those interested in the enormous and burgeoning problem of global antimicrobial resistance and its impact on humans in the twenty-first century, I highly recommend starting with Finland (1955). He published nearly 800 papers in the peer-reviewed medical literature—many of them on antimicrobials and the problems they engendered—during a long and illustrious career in infectious diseases that spanned nearly 55 years and bridged the eras before and following the introduction of antibiotics. His accounts and those of his contemporaries clearly portended our current resistance dilemma.

1. North E. A treatise on a malignant epidemic commonly called spotted fever. New York: T. & J. Swords; 1811.
2. Lesch JE. Conceptual change in an empirical science: the discovery of the first alkaloids. Hist Stud Phys Sci. 1981;11:305–28.
3. Garfield S. Mauve. New York: W. W. Norton and Co.; 2001.
4. Bayer website. http://www.bayer.com/en/history.aspx. Accessed 15 Apr 2012.
5. Lesch JE. The first miracle drugs: how the sulfa drugs transformed medicine. New York: Oxford University Press; 2007. p. 41.
6. Travis AS. The rainbow makers: the origins of the synthetic dyestuffs industry in Western Europe. Bethlehem, PA: Lehigh University Press; 1993.
7. Fairbanks VF. Blue gods, blue oil, and blue people. Mayo Clin Proc. 1994;69:889–92.
8. Jeffreys D. Hell's cartel: I. G. Farben and the making of Hitler's war machine. New York: Henry Holt and CO.; 2008.
9. Sneader W. The discovery of aspirin: a reappraisal. Br Med J. 2000;321:1591–4.
10. Hosztafi S. The history of heroin. Acta Pharm Hung. 2001;71:233–42.
11. Jeffreys D. Hell's cartel: I. G. Farben and the making of Hitler's war machine. New York: Henry Holt and Co; 2008.
12. Parascandola J. The theoretical basis of Paul Ehrlich's chemotherapy. J Hist Med Allied Sci. 1981;36:19–43.
13. Sepkowitz K. One hundred years of Salvarsan. N Engl J Med. 2011;365:291–3.
14. Hager T. The demon under the microscope. New York: Harmony Books; 2006.

15. Nuland SB. Doctors: the biography of medicine. New York: Random House Inc.; 1988. p. 304–42.
16. Hörlein H. The chemotherapy of infectious diseases caused by protozoa and bacteria. Proc R Soc Med. 1936;29:313–24.
17. Crawford E. German scientists and Hitler's vendetta against the Nobel Prizes. Hist Stud Phys Biol Sci. 2000;31:37–53.
18. Long P. Award of the Nobel Prize in Physiology or Medicine to Dr. Gerhard Domagk. The Scientific Monthly. 1940;50:82–4.
19. Borkin J. The crime and punishment of I. G. Farben. New York: MacMillan Publishing Co. Inc.; 1978.
20. Time. "Prontosil", Dec. 28, 1936, vol. 28. p.23.
21. Colebrook L, Kenny M. Treatment of human puerperal infections, and of experimental infections in mice, with Prontosil. Lancet. 1936;227:1279–81.
22. Harding TS. Chemotherapy and Prontosil. Sci Am. 1938;138:28–9.
23. Galdston I. Behind the sulfa drugs: a short history of chemotherapy. New York: D. Appleton-Century Co; 1943.
24. Wax PM. Elixirs, diluents, and the passage of the 1938 Federal Food, Drug and Cosmetic Act. Ann Intern Med. 1995;122:456–61.
25. Schwentker FF, Gelman S, Long PH. The treatment of meningococcic meningitis with sulfanilamide. JAMA. 1937;108:1407–8.
26. Lax E. The mold in Dr. Florey's coat. New York: Henry Holt and Co.; 2005.
27. Austrian R, Gold J. Pneumococcal bacteremia with especial reference to bacteremic Pneumococcal pneumonia. Ann Intern Med. 1964;60:759–76.
28. Darwin C. On the origins of species. New York: Dover Publications; 2006.
29. Carpenter CM, Ackerman H, Winchester HE, Whittle J. Correlation of in vitro sulfonamide resistance of gonococci with results of sulfonamide therapy. Am J Pub Health. 1944;34:250–4.
30. Beigelman PM, Rantz LA. The clinical importance of coagulase-positive, penicillin-resistant *Staphylococcus aureus*. N Engl J Med. 1950;242:353–8.
31. Finland M. Emergence of antibiotic-resistant bacteria. N Engl J Med. 1955;253:909–22, 969–79, 1019–28.
32. Feldman HA. Sulfonamide-resistant meningococci. Annu Rev Med. 1967;18:495–506.
33. Schrag PE, Hamrick FD. An outbreak of meningococcal meningitis in North Carolina caused by sulfonamide-resistant *Neisseria meningitidis*. North Carolina Med J. 1968;29:108–10.
34. Chitwood LA. The prevalence of sulfadiazine resistant meningococci in Oklahoma, 1968. Okla St Med Assoc J. 1969;62:232–5.
35. Alexander CE, Sanborn WR, Cherriere G, Crocker Jr. WH, Ewald PE, Kay CR. Sulfadiazine-resistant group A *Neisseria meningitidis*. Science. 1968;161:1019.
36. Vassiliadis P, Kanellakis A, Papadakis J. Sulphadiazine-resistant group A meningococcal isolated during the 1968 meningitis epidemic in Greece. J Hyg Camb. 1969;67:279–88.

Chapter 7: A Brief History of Vaccines

No history of vaccines would be complete without a thorough discussion of the development of the smallpox vaccine. This must begin with Edward Jenner and his influences and works. Information on his mentor, the great surgeon and physiologist John Hunter, is found in Nuland (1988) and in Hunter's own words (The Royal College of Surgeons of England 1976). Important insights into the traditional rural folklore surrounding smallpox protection are provided in Pead (2009) and Baxby

(2004). Of course, no history of vaccines would also be complete without a thorough history of the "Old Gloucester" breed of cattle, as provided in Stout (1993). Jenner's background is well described in Fisher (1991). Jenner himself (1978) elegantly described the actual case reports and scientific investigation regarding vaccination with cowpox and its protection against smallpox; his *Inquiry* is a must-read for those interested in the history of vaccines. Debré's (1994) biography of Pasteur is an excellent source of information about the great scientist. The original, classic papers of Mayer, Ivanowsky, and Beijerinck from the last years of the nineteenth century make for great reading and are beautifully gathered in a single monograph by the American Phytopathological Society Press (1942). Oshinsky (2005) provides one of the best and most highly readable accounts of the polio vaccine story in its complete and complex dimensions; it is really a social history of America in the early to mid twentieth century. Finally, I refer to my own work, *Vaccines: A Biography* (Artenstein 2009), multiple times throughout this chapter.

1. Turk JL, Allen E. The influence of John Hunter's inoculation practice on Edward Jenner's discovery of vaccination against smallpox. J R Soc Med. 1990;83:266–7.
2. Nuland SB. Doctors: the biography of medicine. New York: Random House Inc.; 1988. pp. 171–99.
3. Royal College of Surgeons of England. Letters from the past: from John Hunter to Edward Jenner. The Stonebridge Press; Bristol, 1976.
4. Artenstein AW. Smallpox. In: Artenstein AW, editor. Vaccines: a biography. New York: Springer; 2009.
5. Stout A. The Old Gloucester: the story of a cattle breed. Gloucester: Gloucester Cattle Society; 1993.
6. Pead PJ. Benjamin Jesty: Dorset's vaccination pioneer. West Sussex: Timefile Books; 2009.
7. Fisher RB. Edward Jenner 1749–1823. London: André Deutsch Limited; 1991.
8. Baxby D. Vaccination: Jenner's legacy. Berkeley: The Jenner Educational Trust; 1994.
9. Jenner E. An inquiry into the causes and effects of the variolae vaccine: a disease discovered in some of the western counties of England, particularly Gloucestershire, and known by the name of the cow pox. Birmingham, AL: The Classics of Medicine Library, Division of Gryphon Editions, Ltd.; 1978.
10. Debré P. Louis Pasteur [English edition: Debré P (1998) Louis Pasteur (E. Forster, trans)]. Baltimore: The Johns Hopkins University Press; 1994.
11. Gheorghiu M, Lagranderie M, Balazuc A-M. Tuberculosis and BCG. In: Artenstein AW, editor. Vaccines: a biography. New York: Springer; 2009.
12. Carpenter CCJ, Hornick RB. Killed vaccines: cholera, typhoid, and plague. In: Artenstein AW, editor. Vaccines: a biography. New York: Springer; 2009.
13. Grabenstein JD. Toxoid vaccines. In: Artenstein AW, editor. Vaccines: a biography. New York: Springer; 2009.
14. Bos L. Beijerinck's work on tobacco mosaic virus: historical context and legacy. Phil Trans R Soc Lond. 1999;354:675–85.
15. Mayer A. Concerning the mosaic disease of tobacco. Die Landwirtschaftliche Versuchsstationen 1886;32:451–67.[English edition: Mayer A (J. Johnson, trans). In: Phytopathological classics. Number 7. St. Paul, MN: American Phytopathological Society Press; 1942. p. 11–24.
16. Ivanowski D. Concerning the mosaic disease of the tobacco plant. St. Petersb Acad Imp Sci Bull. 1892;35:60–7.[English edition: Mayer A (J. Johnson, trans). In: Phytopathological classics. Number 7. St. Paul, MN: American Phytopathological Society Press; 1942. p. 27–30.

17. Beijerinck MW. Concerning a *contagium vivum fluidum* as a cause of the spot-disease of tobacco leaves. Verhandelingen der Koninkyke akademie Wettenschappen te Amsterdam 1898;65:3–21 [English edition: Beijerinck MW (J. Johnson, trans). In: Phytopathological classics. Number 7. St. Paul, MN: American Phytopathological Society Press; 1942. p. 33–52.

18. Artenstein AW. The discovery of viruses: advancing science and medicine by challenging dogma. Int J Infect Dis. 2012; 16:e470–3.

19. Rivers TM. Filterable viruses. J Bacteriol. 1927;14:217–58.

20. Woodruff AM, Goodpasture EW. The susceptibility of the chorio-allantoic membrane of chick embryos to infection with the fowl-pox virus. Am J Pathol. 1931;7:209–22.

21. Artenstein NC, Artenstein AW. The discovery of viruses and the evolution of vaccinology. In: Artenstein AW, editor. Vaccines: a biography. New York: Springer; 2009. p. 141–58.

22. Enders JF, Weller TH, Robbins FC. Cultivation of the Lansing strain of poliomyelitis virus in cultures of various human embryonic tissues. Science. 1949;109:85–7.

23. Oshinsky DM. Polio: an American story. New York: Oxford University Press; 2005.

Chapter 8: That Soluble Specific Substance

Osler's (1893) famous textbook is a good embarkation point for a chapter on the discovery of the immunologic specificity of the polysaccharide capsules of pneumococci and meningococci because in it he devotes substantial space to a discussion of the importance of the pneumococcus and lobar pneumonia in the late nineteenth century. It is worth reading the original scientific descriptions of the work in Dochez (1917), Heidelberger (1923), and Heidelberger (1924). Of course, reading the first and immediately classic description of the "transforming" power of DNA by Avery (1944) and colleagues is a necessity; it not only changed the basis of biology at the time, but it launched the modern molecular era. Dubos (1976) provides a wonderfully personal biography of Oswald Avery from the perspective of someone who was mentored by the man. Kuhn's work (1996) is a provocative discussion of the concept of "paradigm shifts" in thinking in science through the process of innovation, discovery, and the inherent controversies that accompany the process. Although written from the perspective of physical science, the observations apply equally to the biological realm as well as other disciplines. Finally, the reminiscences of Heidelberger (1979) and Kabat (1983) are almost entire autobiographies and give significant insight into the motivations of these two great but not widely appreciated figures in science.

1. Osler W. The principles and practice of medicine. New York: D. Appleton and Co.; 1893.
2. Malkin HM. The trials and tribulations of George Miller Sternberg (1838–1915)—America's first bacteriologist. Perspect Biol Med. 1993;36:666–78.
3. Austrian R. The Jeremiah Metzger lecture: of gold and pneumococci: a history of pneumococcal vaccines in South Africa. Trans Am Clin Climatol Assoc. 1978;89:141–61.
4. Dochez AR, Avery OT. The elaboration of specific soluble substance by pneumococcus during growth. J Exp Med. 1917;26:477–93.

5. MacLeod C. Obituary notice: Oswald Theodore Avery, 1877–1955. J Gen Microbiol. 1957;17:539–49.
6. Avery OT, MacLeod CM, McCarty M. Studies on the chemical nature of the substance inducing transformation of pneumococcal types: inductions of transformation by desoxyribonucleic acid fraction isolated from pneumococcus type III. J Exp Med. 1944;79:137–58.
7. Neufeld F. Ueber die Agglutination der Pneumokokken und über die Theorieen der Agglutination. Z Hyg Infektionskr. 1902;40:54–72.
8. Branham SE. Milestones in the history of the meningococcus. Can J Microbiol. 1956;2:175–88.
9. Dubos RJ. The professor, the institute, and DNA. New York: The Rockefeller University Press; 1976.
10. Heidelberger M, Avery OT. The soluble specific substance of pneumococcus. J Exp Med. 1923;38:73–9.
11. Heidelberger M, Avery OT. The soluble specific substance of pneumococcus. Second paper. J Exp Med. 1924;40:301–17.
12. Kuhn TS. The structure of scientific revolutions. 3rd ed. Chicago: The University of Chicago Press; 1996.
13. Artenstein AW. The discovery of viruses: advancing science and medicine by challenging dogma. Int J Infect Dis. 2012; 16:e470–3
14. Dowling HF. Fighting infection: conquests of the twentieth century. Cambridge: Harvard University Press; MA, 1977.
15. Schiemann O, Casper W. Sind die spezifisch präcipitablen Substanzen der 3 Pneumokokkentypen Haptene? Ztschr f Hyg u Infektionskr. 1927;108:220–57.
16. Finland M, Dowling HF. Cutaneous reactions and antibody response to intracutaneous injections of pneumococcus polysaccharides. J Immunol. 1935;29:285–99.
17. Finland M, Brown JW. Reactions of human subjects to the injection of purified type specific pneumococcus polysaccharides. J Clin Invest. 1938;17:479–88.
18. MacLeod CM, Hodges RG, Heidelberger M, et al. Prevention of pneumococcal pneumonia by immunization with specific capsular polysaccharides. J Exp Med. 1945;82:445–65.
19. Daniels WB. Meningococcal infections. http://history.amedd.army.mil/booksdocs/wwii/infectiousdisvolii/chapter9.htm. Accessed 15 Ap 2012.
20. Woodward TE, ed. The armed forces epidemiological board: the histories of the commissions. Washington DC: Borden Institute; 1994.
21. Heidelberger M. A "pure" organic chemist's downward path: chapter 2—the years at P and S. Annu Rev Biochem. 1979;48:1–21.
22. Kabat EA. Getting started 50 years ago—experiences, perspectives, and problems of the first 21 years. Annu Rev Immunol. 1983;1:1–32.
23. Kabat EA, Kaiser H, Sikorski H. Preparation of the type-specific polysaccharide of the type I meningococcus and a study of its effectiveness as an antigen in human beings. J Exp Med. 1945;80:299–307.
24. Austrian R, Gold J. Pneumococcal bacteremia with especial reference to bacteremic pneumococcal pneumonia. Ann Intern Med. 1964;60:759–76.
25. Artenstein MS, Gold R. Current status of prophylaxis of meningococcal disease. Mil Med. 1970;135:735–9.
26. Artenstein AW. Polysaccharide vaccines. In: Artenstein AW, editor. Vaccines: a biography. New York: Springer; 2009. p. 279–99.

Chapter 9: Towards a Vaccine

The history of Walter Reed Army Medical Center comprises a substantial volume of information relating to American medical history in general, as many advancements in the field in this country derived from the Army Medical Department, beginning with General George Washington's decision to implement force-wide, compulsory smallpox vaccination during the Revolutionary War. Standlee (2009) provides a window into the first 50 years of Walter Reed Hospital's history—one that remained in a file cabinet until it was dusted off and published—without changes to the original manuscript—in 2009, just before the campus was vacated by the military in its move to suburban Maryland. The WRAIR story is both highly compelling and very personal. My father worked there from 1959 to 1961; and again from 1962 to 1976—the latter stint as a civilian. I spent 10 years at Walter Reed, both at the Walter Reed Army Medical Center (WRAMC) and at WRAIR from 1986 to 1996. Writing about its history was cathartic for me. Both Gotschlich and Goldschneider provided important insights into the atmosphere surrounding the meningococcal research; it would have been helpful to have my father's insights, but he died, tragically, in 1976—at the age of 46—from complications of laboratory-acquired hepatitis. The five papers from the WRAIR group—two with Goldschneider as first author and three with Gotschlich as first author—were published in 1969 as a five-paper monograph in the *Journal of Experimental Medicine*, which was extremely unusual at the time. In today's era, the data in these five papers would probably be allocated to at least twice that many publications and would likely trickle out over years. These are considered classics in the field and mandatory reading for anyone interested or working in meningococcal disease. The definitive field trials of the first meningococcal vaccine, Artenstein (1970) and Gold (1971), tell a convincing story of the efficacy of this product in the basic training setting. The "tradition" of self-experimentation in medical research is handled well by Altman (1986). Finally, the atmosphere of Army basic training in the 1960s was informed by multiple sources, including Morton (2004), Rabon (2010), Hasford (1978)—whose semiautobiographical novella served as the basis for Kubrick's film *Full Metal Jacket* a decade later—and my own experiences in officer's basic training supplemented by numerous discussions I had over the years with patients and staff at WRAMC and WRAIR.

1. Borden Institute. Walter Reed Army Medical Center Centennial: a pictorial history 1 909–2009. Washington DC: Office of the Surgeon General; 2009.
2. Standlee MW. Borden's dream. Washington DC: Office of the Surgeon General; 2009.
3. Offit PA. Vaccinated: one man's quest to defeat the world's deadliest diseases. New York: Smithsonian Books; 2007.
4. Brundage JF, Zollinger WD. Evolution of meningococcal disease epidemiology in the U.S. Army. In: Vedros NA, editor. Evolution of meningococcal disease, vol. 1. Boca Raton: CRC Press; 1987.
5. Brown JW, Condit PK. Meningococcal infections: Fort Ord and California. Calif Med. 1965;102:171–180.
6. Parkman PD, Buescher EL, Artenstein MS. Proc Soc Exp Biol Med. 1962;111:225–30.

7. Buescher EL. Malcolm Stewart Artenstein 1930–1976; A recollection of a physician-scientist who contributed his best to the Walter Reed Army Institute of Research as its Chief, Department of Bacterial Diseases, 1966–1976. Memorial Service Address, March 18th, 1976.

8. Buescher EL. Malcolm S. Artenstein, 1930–1976. J Infect Dis. 1976;133:594.

9. Robinson D. The miracle finders. New York: David McKay Co., Inc.; 1976.

10. Interview with Emil Gotschlich, M.D., April 24th, 2012.

11. Interview with Irving Goldschneider, M.D., July 8th, 2009.

12. Goldschneider I, Gotschlich EC, Artenstein MS. Human immunity to the meningococcus. I. The role of humoral antibodies. J Exp Med. 1969;129:1307–26.

13. Goldschneider I, Gotschlich EC, Artenstein MS. Human immunity to the meningococcus. II. Development of natural immunity. J Exp Med. 1969;129:1327–48.

14. Gotschlich EC, Liu TY, Artenstein MS. Human immunity to the meningococcus. III. Preparation and immunochemical properties of the group A, group B, and group C meningococcal polysaccharides. J Exp Med. 1969;129:1349–65.

15. Gotschlich EC, Goldschneider I, Artenstein MS. Human immunity to the meningococcus. IV. Immunogenicity of group A and group C meningococcal polysaccharides in human volunteers. J Exp Med. 1969;129:1367–84.

16. Altman LK. Who goes first? The story of self-experimentation in medicine. New York: Random House; 1986.

17. Gotschlich EC, Goldschneider I, Artenstein MS. Human immunity to the meningococcus. V. The effect of immunization with meningococcal group C polysaccharide on the carrier state. J Exp Med. 1969;129:1385–95.

18. Morton J. Reluctant lieutenant: from Basic to OCS in the sixties. College Station, TX: Texas A&M University Press; 2004.

19. Rabon M. Billy Don, Basic and me. Pennsylvania: Infinity Publishing; 2010.

20. Hasford. G. The short-timers. 1978. Available at: http://www.gustavhasford.com/ST.htm. Accessed 24 Mar 2012.

21. Artenstein MS, Gold R, Zimmerly JG, et al. Prevention of meningococcal disease by group C polysaccharide vaccine. N Engl J Med. 1970;282:417–20.

22. Gold R, Artenstein MS. Meningococcal infections. 2. Field trial of group C meningococcal polysaccharide vaccine in 1969–1970. Bull WHO. 1971;45:279–82.

23. Artenstein MS. Control of meningococcal meningitis with meningococcal vaccines. Yale J Biol Med. 1975;48:197–200.

Chapter 10: Success for Half

The story related to the clinical trials of the meningococcal polysaccharide vaccines in children and infants and the more recent progress on the conjugate vaccine front—over the past two decades—can only really be reconstructed through a thorough reading of the medical literature of the time. The distinct immunology of the group B meningococcus has also been the subject of a considerable volume of scientific literature over the past 40 years, best documented in the original manuscripts.

1. Miller R. Dr. Martin Randolph, 'a giant' of medicine, dead at 92. NewsTimes, Mar 5th, 2010. Available at: http://www.newstimes.com/news/article/Dr-Martin-Randolph-a-giant-of-medicine-dead-393696.php. Accessed 23 Apr 2012).

2. Jacobs W. Danbury's gift to medicine. New York Times, September 28th, 1997. Available at http://www.nytimes.com/1997/09/28/nyregion/danbury-s-gift-to-medicine.html. Accessed 22 Apr 2012.

3. Interview with Martha Lepow, M.D., April 24th, 2012.

4. Goldschneider I, Gotschlich EC, Artenstein MS. Human immunity to the meningococcus. I. The role of humoral antibodies. J Exp Med. 1969;129:1307–26.
5. Interview with Irving Goldschneider, M.D., July 8th, 2009.
6. Goldschneider I, Lepow ML, Gotschlich EC. Immunogenicity of the group A and group C meningococcal polysaccharides in children. J Infect Dis. 1972;125:509–19.
7. de Morais JS, Munford RS, Risi JB, Antezana E, Feldman RA. Epidemic disease due to serogroup C Neisseria meningitidis in Saõ Paulo, Brazil. J Infect Dis. 1974;129:568–71.
8. Taunay A de E, Galvao PA, de Morais JS, Gotschlich EC, Feldman RA. Disease prevention by meningococcal serogroup C polysaccharide vaccine in preschool children: results after eleven months in Saõ Paulo, Brazil. Pediatr Res. 1974;8:429.
9. Erwa HH, Haseeb MA, Idris AA, Lapeyssonnie L, Sanborn WR, Sippel JE. A serogroup A meningococcal polysaccharide vaccine: studies in the Sudan to combat cerebrospinal meningitis caused by Neisseria meningitidis group A. Bull WHO. 1973;49:301–5.
10. Wahdan MH, Rizk F, El-Akkad AM, et al. A controlled field trial of a serogroup A meningococcal polysaccharide vaccine. Bull WHO. 1973;48:667–73.
11. Mäkelä PH, Käyhty H, Weckström P, Sivonen A, Renkonen O-K. Effect of group-A meningococcal vaccine in Army recruits in Finland. The Lancet. 1975;2:883–6.
12. Gold R, Lepow ML, Goldschneider I, Draper TL, Gotschlich EC. Clinical evaluation of group A and group C meningococcal polysaccharide vaccines in infants. J Clin Invest. 1975;56:1536–47.
13. Stevenson LG. Nobel Prize winners in medicine and physiology 1901–1950. New York: Henry Schuman; 1953.
14. Corner GW. A history of the Rockefeller Institute 1901–1953. New York: The Rockefeller Institute Press; 1964.
15. Artenstein AW. Polysaccharide vaccines. In: Artenstein AW, ed. Vaccines: a biography, New York: Springer; 2009. p. 279–99.
16. Robbins JB, Schneerson R, Anderson P, Smith DH. Prevention of systemic infections, especially meningitis, caused by Haemophilus influenzae type b. JAMA. 1996;276:1181–5.
17. Kyaw MH, Lynfield R, Schaffner W, et al. Effect of introduction of the pneumococcal conjugate vaccine on drug-resistant Streptococcus pneumoniae. N Engl J Med. 2006;354:1455–63.
18. Harrison LH, Trotter CL, Ramsay ME. Global epidemiology of meningococcal disease. Vaccine. 2009;27:B51-63.
19. Wyle FA, Artenstein MS, Brandt BL, et al. Immunologic response of man to group B meningococcal polysaccharide vaccines. J Infect Dis. 1972;126:514–22.
20. Kasper DL, Winkelhake JL, Zollinger WD, Brandt BL, Artenstein MS. Immunochemcial similarity between polysaccharide antigens of Escherichia coli 07:K1(L):NM and group B Neisseria meningitidis. J Immunol. 1973;110:262–68.
21. Finne J, Leinonen M, Makela PH. Antigenic similarities between brain components and bacteria causing meningitis. Implications for vaccine development and pathogenesis. Lancet. 1983;2:355–7.
22. Lo H, Tang CM, Exley RM. Mechanisms of avoidance of host immunity by Neisseria meningitidis and its effect on vaccine development. Lancet Infect Dis. 2009;9:418–27.

Chapter 11: The Future of a Killer

The strategies related to resolving the two major impediments to future, worldwide control and prevention of epidemic meningococcal meningitis—group B meningococci and the problem of epidemic group A disease in the African "meningitis belt"—are most thoroughly described in the original medical literature, much of which has been published over the past decade.

1. Harrison LH, Trotter CL, Ramsay ME. Global epidemiology of meningococcal disease. Vaccine. 2009;27:B51–63.
2. Campbell H, Borrow R, Salisbury D, Miller E. Meningococcal C conjugate vaccine: the experience in England and Wales. Vaccine. 2009;27:B20–9.
3. Poland GA. Prevention of meningococcal disease: current use of polysaccharide and conjugate vaccines. Clin Infect Dis. 2010;50;S45–53.
4. Tan LKK, Carlone GM, Borrow R. Advances in the development of vaccines against *Neisseria meningitidis*. N Engl J Med. 2010;362:1511–20.
5. Pizza M, Scarlato V, Masignani V, et al. Identification of vaccine candidates against serogroup B meningococcus by whole genome sequencing. Science. 2000;287:1816–20.
6. Gossger N, Snape MD, Yu L-M, et al. Immunogenicity and tolerability of recombinant serogroup B meningococcal vaccine administered with or without routine infant vaccinations according to different immunization schedules. JAMA. 2012;307:573–82.
7. PATH: a catalyst for global health. Available at: http://www.path.org/about/index.php. Accessed 30 Apr 2012.
8. Interview with F. Marc LaForce, M.D., May 2nd, 2012.
9. LaForce FM, Konde K, Viviani S, Prézioso M-P. The meningitis vaccine project. Vaccine. 2007;25S:A97–100.
10. Sow SO, Okoko BJ, Diallo A, et al. Immunogenicity and safety of a meningococcal A conjugate vaccine in Africans. N Engl J Med. 2011;364:2293–304.
11. MenAfriVac™ reaches three new African countries. Available at: http://www.meningvax.org. Accessed 3 May 2012.
12. Interview with Paul Offit, M.D., April 25th, 2012.

Selected Bibliography

Altman LK. Who goes first? The story of self-experimentation in medicine. New York: Random House; 1986.

Artenstein AW, editor. Vaccines: a biography. New York: Springer; 2009.

Artenstein MS, Gold R, Zimmerly JG, et al. Prevention of meningococcal disease by group C polysaccharide vaccine. N Engl J Med. 1970;282:417–20.

Austrian R. Random gleanings from a life with the pneumococcus. J Infect Dis. 1975;131: 474–84.

Austrian R, Gold J. Pneumococcal bacteremia with especial reference to bacteremic pneumococcal pneumonia. Ann Intern Med. 1964;60:759–76.

Bäumler E. Paul Ehrlich: scientist for life [G. Edwards, trans]. New York: Holmes & Meier; 1984.

Baxby D. Vaccination: Jenner's Legacy. Berkeley: The Jenner Educational Trust; 1994.

Berkeley MJ. Observations, botanical and physiological, on the Potato Murrain. J Hortic Soc Lond. 1846;1:9–34.

Bliss M. William Osler: a life in medicine. New York: Oxford University Press; 1999.

Borkin J. The crime and punishment of I.G. Farben. New York: Macmillan Publishing Co., Inc.; 1978.

Brock TD. Robert Koch: a life in medicine and bacteriology. Washington, DC: ASM Press; 1988.

Brown RE. Rockefeller medicine men: medicine and capitalism in America. Berkeley: University of California Press; 1979.

Buczacki S. Presidential address, Linnean Society of London: Berkeley's legacy—who cares? Mycol Res. 2001;105(11):1283–94.

Bulloch W. The history of bacteriology: University of London Heath Clark Lectures, 1936. New York: Dover Publications, Inc.; 1938.

Bynum WF. Science and the practice of medicine in the nineteenth century. New York: Cambridge University Press; 1994.

Cantor NF. In the wake of the plague: the black death and the world it made. New York: Perennial; 2002.

Carpenter CC. The Jeremiah Metzger Lecture. Myths, mandarins and molecules: the cautionary tale of cholera. Trans Am Clin Climatol Assoc. 1981;92:167–93.

Chernow R. Titan: the life of John D. Rockefeller, Sr. New York: Random House Inc.; 1998.

Conrad LI, Neve M, Nutton V, Porter R, Wear A. The western medical tradition 800 BC to AD 1800. New York: Cambridge University Press; 1995.

Cook ND. Born to die: disease and New World Conquest, 1492–1650. Cambridge: Cambridge University Press; 1998.

Corner GW. A history of the Rockefeller Institute 1901–1953. New York: The Rockefeller Institute Press; 1964.

Councilman WT, Mallory FB, Wright JH. Epidemic cerebro-spinal meningitis and its relation to other forms of meningitis. Boston: Report of the State Board of Health of MA; 1898. p. 1–178.

Danielson L, Mann E. The history of a singular and very mortal disease, which lately made its appearance in Medfield—symptoms of the disorder—its progress and termination—appearances on dissection—the different methods of treatment, and what eventually proved successful. Med Agric Reg. 1806;1:65–9.

Darwin C. On the origins of species by means of natural selection. London: John Murray; 1859.

Debré P. Louis Pasteur [E. Forster, trans]. Baltimore: The Johns Hopkins University Press; 1998.

Diamond J. Guns, germs, and steel: the fates of human societies. New York: W. W. Norton & Company; 1997.

Dobell C. Antony van Leeuwenhoek and his "Little Animals": being some account of the Father of Protozoology and Bacteriology and his multifarious discoveries in these disciplines. New York: Dover Publications, Inc.; 1960.

Dowling HF. Fighting infection: conquests of the twentieth century. Cambridge: Harvard University Press; 1977.

Dubos R, Dubos J. The white plague. Boston: Little Brown; 1956.

Finland M. Emergence of antibiotic-resistant Bacteria. N Engl J Med. 1955;253:909–22, 969–79, 1019–28.

Fisher RM. Edward Jenner 1749–1823. London: André Deutsch Limited; 1991.

Flexner JT. An American Saga: the story of Helen Thomas and Simon Flexner. London: Fordham University Press; 1993.

Flexner S. The results of the serum treatment in thirteen hundred cases of epidemic meningitis. J Exp Med. 1913;15:553–75.

Flexner S, Flexner JT. William Henry Welch and the heroic age of American medicine. New York: Viking Press; 1941.

Fracastorius H. Contagion, contagious diseases and their treatment [W.C. Wright, trans]. New York: G.P. Putnam's Sons; 1930.

Galdston I. Behind the sulfa drugs: a short history of chemotherapy. New York: D. Appleton-Century Co; 1943.

Garfield S. Mauve. New York: W. W. Norton and Co.; 2001.

Geison GL. The private science of Louis Pasteur. Princeton: Princeton University Press; 1995.

Gold R, Artenstein MS. Meningococcal infections. 2. Field trial of group C meningococcal polysaccharide vaccine in 1969–1970. Bull WHO. 1971;45:279–82.

Goldschneider I, Gotschlich EC, Artenstein MS. Human immunity to the meningococcus. I. The role of humoral antibodies. J Exp Med. 1969a;129:1307–26.

Goldschneider I, Gotschlich EC, Artenstein MS. Human immunity to the meningococcus. II. Development of natural immunity. J Exp Med. 1969b;129:1327–48.

Gotschlich EC, Goldschneider I, Artenstein MS. Human immunity to the meningococcus. III. Preparation and immunochemical properties of the group A, group B, and group C meningococcal polysaccharides. J Exp Med. 1969a;129:1349–65.

Gotschlich EC, Goldschneider I, Artenstein MS. Human immunity to the meningococcus. IV. Immunogenicity of group A and group C meningococcal polysaccharides in human volunteers. J Exp Med. 1969b;129:1367–84.

Gotschlich EC, Goldschneider I, Artenstein MS. Human immunity to the meningococcus. V. The effect of immunization with meningococcal group C polysaccharide on the carrier state. J Exp Med. 1969c;129:1385–95.

Gram C. The differential staining of schizomycetes in tissue sections and in dried preparations. In: Brock TD, editor. Milestones in microbiology: 1546 to 1940 [T.D. Brock, trans]. Washington, DC: ASM Press; 1999. p. 215–8.

Greenwood B. 100 Years of epidemic meningitis in West Africa—has anything changed? Trop Med Int Health. 2006;11:773–80.

Hager T. The demon under the microscope: from battlefield hospitals to Nazi Labs, one doctors heroic search for the world's first miracle drug. New York: Harmony Books; 2006.

Harding-Rains AJ. Joseph Lister and antisepsis. Sussex: Priory Press; 1977.

Hasford G. The short-timers. 1978. Available at: http://www.gustavhasford.com/ST.htm

Hempel S. The strange case of the broad street pump: John Snow and the mystery of cholera. Berkeley, CA: University of California Press; 2007.

Herr M. Dispatches. New York: Avon Books; 1978.

Hopkins DR. The greatest killer: smallpox in history. Chicago: University of Chicago Press; 1983.

Jeffreys D. Hell's Cartel: I. G. Farben and the making of Hitler's war machine. New York: Henry Holt and Co.; 2008.

Jenner E. An inquiry into the causes and effects of the variolae vaccine: a disease discovered in some of the western counties of England, particularly Gloucestershire, and known by the name of the cow pox. Birmingham, AL: The Classics of Medicine Library, Division of Gryphon Editions, Ltd.; 1978.

Johnson S. The ghost map: the story of London's most terrifying epidemic—and how it changed science, cities, and the modern world. New York: Riverhead Books; 2006.

Koch R. The etiology of anthrax, based on the life history of *Bacillus anthracis*. In: Brock TD, editor. Milestones in microbiology: 1546 to 1940 [T.D. Brock, trans]. Washington, DC: ASM Press; 1999. p. 89–95.

Lapeyssonnie L. La Méningite Cérébro-spinale en Afrique. Bull World Health Organ. 1963;28(Suppl):1–114.

Latham RG. The works of Thomas Sydenham, M.D. [translated from the Latin Edition of Dr. Greenhill with a life of the author]. London: C. and J. Adlard, Printers; 1848.

Lax E. The mold in Dr. Florey's coat. New York: Henry Holt and Co.; 2005.

Lesch JE. The first miracle drugs: how the sulfa drugs transformed medicine. New York: Oxford University Press; 2007. p. 41.

Ligon BL. Albert Ludwig Sigesmund Neisser: discover of the cause of gonorrhea. Semin Pediatr Infect Dis. 2005;16:336–41.

Lister J. On a new method of treating compound fracture, abscess, and so forth; with observations on the conditions of suppuration. In: Brock TD, editor. Milestones in microbiology: 1546 to 1940 [T.D. Brock, trans]. Washington, DC: ASM Press; 1999. p. 83–5.

Major RH. Classic descriptions of disease: with biographical sketches of the authors. 3rd ed. Springfield: Charles C. Thomas; 1945.

McCarty M. The transforming principle: discovering that genes are made of DNA. New York: W. W. Norton and Co.; 1985.

McCullough D. The path between the seas: the creation of the Panama Canal 1870–1914. New York: Simon and Shuster; 1977.

McNeill WH. Plagues and people. New York: Doubleday; 1976.

Money NP. The triumph of the fungi: a rotten history. New York: Oxford University Press; 2007.

Morton J. Reluctant lieutenant: from Basic to OCS in the sixties. College Station, TX: Texas A&M University Press; 2004.

North E. A treatise on a malignant epidemic commonly called spotted fever. New York: T. & J. Swords; 1811.

Nuland SB. Doctors: the biography of medicine. New York: Random House Inc.; 1988.

Nuland SB. The doctors' plague: germs, childbed fever, and the strange story of Ignác Semmelweis. New York: W.W. Norton & Company; 2003.

Offit PA. Vaccinated: one man's quest to defeat the world's deadliest diseases. New York: Smithsonian Books; 2007.

Oliver WW. The man who lived for tomorrow. New York: E.P. Dutton and Co., Inc; 1941.

Oshinsky D. Polio: an american story. New York: Oxford University Press; 2005.

Osler W. The Cavendish lecture on the etiology and diagnosis of cerebro-spinal fever. Br Med J. 1899;1:1517–28.

Panum PL. Observations made during the epidemic of measles on the Faroe Islands in the year 1846 [Delta Omega Society, trans]. New York: American Public Health Association; 1940.

Parascandola J. The theoretical basis of Paul Ehrlich's chemotherapy. J Hist Med Allied Sci. 1981;36:19–43.

Pasteur L. On the organized bodies which exist in the atmosphere; examination of the doctrine of spontaneous generation. In: Brock TD, editor. Milestones in microbiology: 1546 to 1940 [T.D. Brock, trans]. Washington, DC: ASM Press; 1999. p. 43–8.

Pead PJ. Benjamin Jesty: Dorset's vaccination pioneer. West Sussex: Timefile Books; 2009.

Peters FE. The Hajj: the Muslim pilgrimage to Mecca and the holy places. Princeton, NJ: Princeton University Press; 1994.

Quétel C. The history of syphilis [J. Braddock and P. Brian, trans]. Baltimore, MD: The Johns Hopkins University Press; 1992.

Rabon M. Billy Don, Basic and me. Pennsylvania: Infinity Publishing; 2010.

Redi of Aresso F. Experiments on the generation of insects [Mab Bigelow, trans]. Chicago: The Open Court Publishing Company; 1909.

Robinson D. The miracle finders. New York: David McKay Co., Inc.; 1976.

Royal College of Surgeons of England. Letters from the past: from John Hunter to Edward Jenner. Bristol: The Stonebridge Press; 1976.

Silverman M. Magic in a bottle. New York: The Macmillian Company; 1948.

Snow J. On the mode of communication of cholera. London: Churchill; 1855.

Standlee M. Borden's dream. Washington, DC: Bordon Institute, Office of the Surgeon General, US Army; 2009.

Steiner PE. Disease in the civil war: natural biological warfare in 1861–1865. Springfield, IL: Charles C. Thomas Publisher; 1968.

Stevenson LG. Nobel prize winners in medicine and physiology 1901–1950. New York: Henry Schuman; 1953.

Stout A. The old Gloucester: the story of a cattle breed. Gloucester: Gloucester Cattle Society; 1993.

Sydenham T. The works of Thomas Sydenham, M.D. on Acute and chronic diseases: wherein their histories and modes of cure, as recited by him, are delivered with accuracy and perspicuity. To which are Subjoined notes, corrective and explanatory, from the most eminent. 1788th ed. London: G.G.H. and J. Robinson, W. Otridge, S. Hayes, and E. Newbery; 1788.

Taylor FS. The conquest of bacteria. New York: The Philosophical Library; 1942.

Tracey KJ. Fatal sequence: the killer within. New York: Dana Press; 2006.

Travis AS. The rainbow makers: the origins of the synthetic dyestuffs industry in Western Europe. Bethlehem, PA: Lehigh University Press; 1993.

van Leeuwenhoek A. Microscopical observations about animals in the scurf of the teeth. In: Brock TD, editor. Milestones in microbiology: 1546 to 1940 [T.D. Brock, trans]. Washington, DC: ASM Press; 1999. p. 9–11.

Vieusseux G. Mémoire sur la Maladie qui a Regné à Genève au Printemps de 1805. J Med Chi Pharm. 1805;11:163–93.

Weichselbaum A. Ueber die Aetiologie der Akuten Menigitis Cerebro-spinalis. Fortschr Med. 1887;5(18):573–83.

Zinsser H. Rats, lice and history. Boston: Little, Brown and Company; 1934.

Acknowledgments

I wish to thank Dr. David Greer, Dean Emeritus at Brown Medical School and a mentor, friend, and colleague of mine for the last decade and Dr. Steven Opal, Chief of Infectious Diseases at Memorial Hospital, Professor of Medicine at Brown, and a great friend, colleague, and collaborator for many years. They both graciously read multiple drafts of this work and provided helpful critiques and insights that improved the final product. I also wish to thank Kathy Bollesen and Margo Katz who, as always, provided outstanding administrative support. They continue to be reliable and helpful after all these years. Finally, I want to acknowledge the infectious diseases researchers at the Walter Reed Army Institute of Research during the 1960s and 1970s—my father's time—and during the latter 1980s and 1990s—my time there. Even after nearly 2 decades, the memories are vivid and compelling. I can clearly recall the sights, sounds, smells, and sense of that highly charged, intellectual atmosphere, and—at times—I still marvel at all that was accomplished within the eccentric, "Catch-22" subtext that permeated the place. These feelings evoke a strong sense of nostalgia for the great people that worked there and the great work they did.

A.W. Artenstein, *In the Blink of an Eye: The Deadly Story of Epidemic Meningitis*,   129
DOI 10.1007/978-1-4614-4845-7, © Springer Science+Business Media New York 2013

Subject Index

Name Index

A.W. Artenstein, *In the Blink of an Eye: The Deadly Story of Epidemic Meningitis*,
DOI 10.1007/978-1-4614-4845-7, © Springer Science+Business Media New York 2013

Printed by Publishers' Graphics LLC
SO20130212.19.22.44